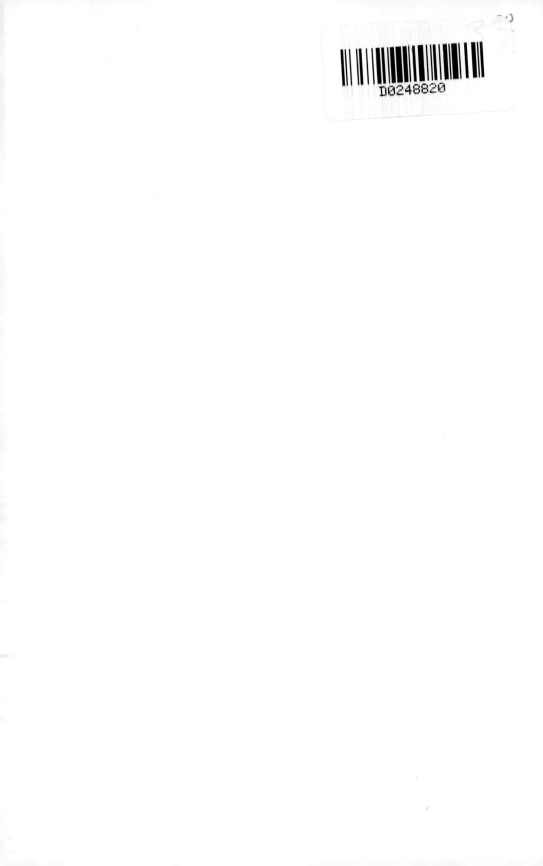

Medical Marriages

Medical Marriages

Edited by

Glen O. Gabbard, M.D.

Section Chief, C. F. Menninger Memorial Hospital;
Staff Psychoanalyst, The Menninger Clinic;
Faculty, Topeka Institute for Psychoanalysis and
Karl Menninger School of Psychiatry
and Mental Health Sciences

and

Roy W. Menninger, M.D.

President and Chief Executive Officer,
The Menninger Foundation, Topeka, Kansas;
Clinical Professor of Psychiatry,
University of Kansas Medical Center (Wichita, Kansas);
Director, Physicians and Their Families Workshop
(Estes Park, Colorado)

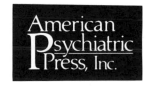

American Psychiatric Press, Inc.

1400 K Street, N.W.
Washington, DC 20005

Copyright © 1988 American Psychiatric Press, Inc.
ALL RIGHTS RESERVED
Manufactured in the United States of America
First Edition
91 92 4 3

Library of Congress Cataloging-in-Publication Data

Medical marriages / edited by Glen O. Gabbard and Roy W.
Menniger.
       p.   cm.
    Bibilography: p.
    Includes index.
    ISBN 0-88048-260-5
    1. Physicians—Family relationships.   2. Marriage.
3. Interpersonal relations.   I. Gabbard, Glen O.
II. Menninger. Roy W., 1926–
    [DNLM: 1. Interpersonal Relations.   2. Marital
Therapy.   3. Marriage.   4. Physicians—psychology.
W 62 M4893]
R707.2.M43 1988
610.69′6—dc19
DNLM/DLC
for Library of Congress   88-14653
                                                        CIP

To our wives,
Joyce and Bev

Contents

Contributors

Lolafaye Coyne, Ph.D., Director, Statistical Laboratory; Associate Director, Hospital Research, The Menninger Clinic, Topeka, Kansas

Glen O. Gabbard, M.D., Section Chief, C. F. Menninger Memorial Hospital; Staff Psychoanalyst, The Menninger Clinic; Faculty, Topeka Institute for Psychoanalysis and Karl Menninger School of Psychiatry and Mental Health Sciences

Stephen A. Jones, M.S.W., Director, Marriage and Family Therapy Training Program; Associate Dean of the Extension Division, Karl Menninger School of Psychiatry and Mental Health Sciences, The Menninger Clinic, Topeka, Kansas

Martin Leichtman, Ph.D., Director of Psychology, Children's Division, The Menninger Clinic, Topeka, Kansas

Bev Menninger, writer, speaker, artist, author

Roy W. Menninger, M.D., President and Chief Executive Officer, The Menninger Foundation, Topeka, Kansas; Clinical Professor of Psychiatry, University of Kansas Medical Center (Wichita, Kansas); Director, Physicians and Their Families Workshop (Estes Park, Colorado)

Carol C. Nadelson, M.D., Associate Psychiatrist-in-Chief, Director, Training and Education, Department of Psychiatry, New England Medical Center Hospitals; Professor and Vice-Chairman, Department of Psychiatry, Tufts University, Boston, Massachusetts

Malkah T. Notman, M.D., Supervising and Training Analyst, Boston Psychoanalytic Institute; Clinical Professor of Psychiatry, Tufts University, Boston, Massachusetts

Domeena C. Renshaw, M.D., Professor of Psychiatry, Loyola University Stritch School of Medicine, Maywood, Illinois

Acknowledgments

The authors gratefully acknowledge permission to reprint portions of the following material:

Chapter 2
Gabbard, G.O., Menninger, R.W., and Coyne, L. "Sources of Conflict in the Medical Marriage." *American Journal of Psychiatry*, 144(5):567–572, 1987. Copyright 1987, the American Psychiatric Association. Portions reprinted by permission.

Chapter 3
Gabbard, G. "The Role of Compulsiveness in the Normal Physician." *Journal of the American Medical Association*, 254(20):2926–2929, 1985. Portions reprinted with permission.

Chapter 5
Menninger, Bev. "The Woman Behind the Man." *The Ladies' Home Journal*, July 1982. Copyright 1982, Meredith Corporation. All Rights Reserved. Portions reprinted from *Ladies' Home Journal* magazine with permission of the author.

Chapter 12
Herbert, A. "The Snake: A Parable." *The CoEvolution Quarterly*, 13:51, March 27, 1977. Reprinted with permission of the author.

Introduction

The original impetus for this book dates back to 1977, when the Department of Continuing Education of The Menninger Clinic began an annual 6-day summer workshop for "Physicians and Their Families" at Estes Park, Colorado, under the initial leadership of Erwin Janssen, M.D., and, for the last 9 years, Roy W. Menninger, M.D. Over the 10 years that these workshops have been held, a steady stream of physicians and their spouses trekked to the mountains of Colorado to speak together and with us about the pleasures and problems of the physician's family life. Despite varying backgrounds in terms of specialization and location of practice, these couples describe remarkably similar concerns about the tasks of balancing the demands of a medical career with the needs of family life.

In a typical workshop week some 20 to 30 couples arrive on a Sunday afternoon and leave the following Friday afternoon. During the 6-day experience, the couples hear lectures on the psychology of the physician, on the nature of marriage, on family systems theory, on the stresses met by the physician's spouse, on the children of medical marriages, and on the sources of conflict in medical marriages. Interspersed with the lectures are regular small group meetings of approximately 90 minutes' duration, in which groups of four to seven couples share their concerns, facilitated by a husband–wife faculty couple that stays with the group all week. These small group discussions are often powerful experiences for the couples as they realize that they are not alone in their struggles and that there are ways to improve communication, to balance the demands of work and family in a reasonably satisfying manner, and to grow and change constructively together.

Several of the contributors to this book have been faculty members at the Estes Park workshops. Although our experiences with couples there serve as one source of data for this book, the data base for this volume is not limited to these workshops. The authors have also drawn on clinical work with physicians who were patients. These patients have turned to some of the authors for marital consultation and therapy, family therapy, sex therapy, individual psychotherapy, and psychoanalysis. Chapter 2 is based on a formal questionnaire study that surveyed a large percentage of the workshop participants. The findings from this study constitute another important data base on which the authors draw. Another source of information that has undoubtedly contributed to the material in this book stems from informal contacts with medical colleagues over the years whose personal and marital despair could not go unnoticed.

This book is not another contribution to the study of the impaired physician. For the most part, the marriages we examine here do not involve a drug- or alcohol-abusing physician or one who is seriously depressed or suicidal. The focus of our attention is the normal physician and the normal medical marriage. *Normality* is a term that has varying usage. For the purposes of this study, we use *normal* to refer to a statistical norm, that is, the typical, average physician and his or her marriage. These are physicians and spouses who function effectively on a day-to-day basis and who are not characterized by serious psychiatric illness. For these "statistically ordinary" physicians, the marriage is a psychological segment of the practice itself. Although it is the principal support system for most physicians, it is at the same time a common source of stress and distress in the life of the typical physician.

Chapter 1 reviews the literature relevant to issues in physician marriages and attempts to define what we see as the major source of conflict among medical couples—namely, the psychological characteristics of most physicians. In this respect we depart from conventional wisdom, which has ascribed the special stresses of the medical marriage to a lack of time because of the inordinate demands of practice and the physician's consequent absence from home.

Chapter 2 reports the results of our formal survey and lends support to our central thesis, that the lack of time is a prominent symptom and not the primary cause of stress in the medical marriage.

Chapter 3 describes the central psychological features of physicians as we see them and our observations of their impact on the typical physician's marriage.

While the marital concerns of physician couples are strikingly similar across a broad cross section of medical marriages, variations do result in different manifestations of the problems. For example, the traditional marriage of a male physician and a female homemaker illustrates characteristic patterns of conflict that will be different from those of the dual-physician marriage, or the single-physician marriage in which the physician is female. The patterns of the "traditional marriage" are the focus of Chapter 4.

Chapter 5, written by Bev Menninger, offers a frank perspective of one medical wife about the need for a separate, "noncontingent" identity, a point of view that is often omitted in collections of writings on this subject.

If the physician is female, characteristic patterns of stress and discord are likely to surface. Because of the psychology of the female physician and the particular stresses on her and her marriage as a result of social and cultural forces, these patterns are different from those of the traditional marriage. These issues are the subjects of Chapters 6 and 7 by Drs. Malkah Notman and Carol Nadelson.

There is remarkably little written about the sexual problems of physician couples. While one might assume that this paucity is related to a high level of sophisticated knowledge about sexual matters on the part of physicians, Domeena Renshaw's extensive work with physician couples does not confirm this assumption. In Chapter 8 Dr. Renshaw provides us with an illuminating discussion of the sexual problems in medical marriages. Her data from years of clinical experience are published here for the first time.

Chapter 9 examines the impact of the physician's marital relationship on the children in the medical marriage. Dr. Martin Leichtman traces the development of the physician's child through each major phase of infancy, childhood, and adolescence.

In Chapter 10 our focus is on adult developmental phases, as we examine the long-term consequences of the physician's psychological characteristics and his or her spouse's response to those characteristics. While the midlife transition is a difficult time for virtually everyone, certain aspects of the medical marriage contribute to special conflictual patterns for the physician and spouse during middle age.

The conflicts inherent in the physician's marital relationship may lead the couple to seek help from marital therapy. In Chapter 11 Steve Jones and Glen Gabbard discuss common complaints that marital therapists hear from physician couples who come for treatment. They also outline therapeutic strategies that are intended to help couples in distress.

The final chapter of the book emphasizes prevention rather than treatment. Here we discuss what couples can do to cope with the stresses inherent in the medical marriage. Just as the marital relationship requires nurturing and attention, so do the individual members of the couple. In Chapter 12 we outline suggestions for responsible behavior both toward oneself and toward one's spouse.

This book is the result of many years of learning from our colleagues; we owe a debt of gratitude to the many physician couples who have had the courage to share some of their deepest fears and concerns with us. We also wish to acknowledge the contributions of the many faculty members who assisted us in those workshops over the years, including Martin and Luisa Leichtman, Steve and Pat Jones, Joe and Patricia Hyland, and Dick and Anna Mae Bollinger. The superb editorial assistance of Mr. James Bakalar greatly improved the book's readability. We also wish to express our deep appreciation to Mrs. Faye Schoenfeld, who spent many long hours typing and organizing our manuscript through a myriad of drafts. Mr. Brent Menninger provided valuable assistance in the data collection process of our questionnaire survey.

Most of all, we are grateful to our wives, Joyce Davidson Gabbard and Bev Menninger, for their patience and understanding, as well as for their substantive contributions throughout the evolution and preparation of this project. They have been our major support system and primary source of inspiration for all that follows.

Glen O. Gabbard, M.D.
Roy W. Menninger, M.D.

The Impossible Dream

Roy W. Menninger, M.D.
Glen O. Gabbard, M.D.

To Be a Doctor

Becoming a physician is a dream many young people acquire early and nourish assiduously through the distractions of childhood, the vicissitudes of adolescence, the demands of college science courses, and the trials of a seemingly endless medical education. It is not only future physicians who are devoted to the dream and its promises. Parents proudly speak of "my son/daughter, the doctor"; lovers make no secret of their beloved's prospects; and spouses express great confidence and high hopes for the future with their physician-mate.

One source of this dream is the image of the physician as a powerful, prestigious, and caring figure who heals (Wilson and Larson 1981; Zabarenko et al. 1970). The dream often begins in childhood experiences. It is both a hope and wish *to be* a prestigious, caring person, and a wish *to do*, to relieve pain and disability, even to vanquish disease and death. The dream is a compound of reality (however idealized), unconscious drives, and compelling social expectations. Its social roots lie in the conception of the physician as a person with a special mission who performs priestly, shamanistic, or apostolic functions (Zabarenko et al. 1970). The helplessness of patients and their dependence on the physician's expertise make them attribute almost magical powers to this shamanistic figure. That gives the physician a social sanction to invade personal privacy to an extent unparalleled in any other profession, and even to invade the body itself.

Social attitudes and the expectations of the medical profession reinforce this dream, even as the disappointment of many patients undermines it. It persists in the face of continuing challenges because it has deep roots in early family life and private fantasy, which are protected from easy scrutiny by unconscious repression.

The Dream Meets Reality

The competing realities of medical practice and marriage expose the limits of what we have called in our chapter title the impossible dream. Any dream, no doubt, expresses wishes that are in part unrealistic. In his pioneering work on the psychology of dreaming, Freud (1900/1962) noted that one of its basic functions is to fulfill repressed childhood wishes that cannot be realized in the external world. Indeed, the medical dream, launched on the voyage of life, brimming with high expectations and fantasies of glorious achievement, often flounders and stagnates in the seas of harsh reality.

Medical education is a "rite of passage" on the way to becoming a member of the medical priesthood, and like any good initiation, it reinforces the novice's faith in the central tenet of the religion: that with enough work, dedication, knowledge, and skill, suffering *can* be alleviated, disease *can* be overcome, and even death defeated. In short, that the impossible *can* be achieved. Ultimately, physicians must learn that cures are exceptional and death can only be delayed. Because they are usually able only to moderate suffering and alleviate distress, they often feel that they have somehow failed, and respond by spending more time learning more, trying harder, working longer. This reflects important unconscious drives and needs, to which we return in more detail in Chapter 3.

The spouse's dreams are at risk as well. The physician partner's total commitment to medical practice spells disappointment for hopes of an intimate marriage. This disillusionment was poignantly described by a physician's wife who participated in our questionnaire study (discussed further in Chapter 2):

> My dream was always that my husband would be my best friend, the one to share all with, and I started our marriage that way. After 1 year of courtship and about 5 years of marriage, I finally realized I was the only one with the expectation and that all my sharing and talking and feeling was falling on deaf ears. So I stopped trying. I realize now I should have ended the marriage,

but I didn't and now it's too late. I'm not the same self-confident person I was when I got married. Now I'm old, fat, and have no job skills. I couldn't support myself—let alone my children. Obviously my self-esteem is low. So I fill my days with volunteer work and the children's activities. I have many women friends, but the conversation never gets too deep. I'm apprehensive as menopause and old age approach. I wonder if I'll be able to handle it emotionally.

Much has been written about the nature and fate of the medical marriage—its features (Schoicket 1978; Taubman 1974); its dynamics (Nelson 1978; Shortt 1979); its natural history (Gerber 1983); its impact on the health of both physician and spouse (Miles et al. 1975); and its relationship to the stresses of medical practice (Coombs 1971; Elliot 1979; Garvey and Tuason 1979; Gerber 1983; McCue 1982; Rhoads 1977; Shaw 1985; Vaillant et al. 1972). Authors have variously accounted for its special characteristics by pointing to the medical education (Gerber 1983; Taubman 1974); the histrionic, dependent nature of the medical wife (Nelson 1978; Shortt 1979; Zemon-Gass and Nichols 1975); the demands of medical practice itself; and the physician's lack of time for the spouse and family (Coombs 1971; Crawford and Lorch 1981; Elliot 1979; Evans 1965; Shortt 1979). Descriptions of the frustrated, loyal, uncomplaining doctor's wife are especially eloquent (Smith 1980; Wolf 1978). A review of the literature suggests that doctors have more than their fair share of marital unhappiness. In a longitudinal prospective study, Vaillant et al. (1972) found much more discord in physicians' marriages than in those of matched controls. Nearly half the doctors in their sample had an unstable marriage; many had considered divorce or had unsatisfying sexual relations. This report is particularly noteworthy since the population studied was skewed in the direction of psychological health. Nevertheless, studies by Garvey and Tuason (1979) and by Rose and Rosow (1972) reveal that divorce is less common than average among physicians. Physician couples are apparently willing to tolerate more marital tension than most. This is confirmed by our own questionnaire survey described in Chapter 2. One physician, when asked if he would seriously consider separating from or divorcing his wife, responded: "Murder, yes! Divorce, no!" A physician's spouse, asked how many times she had been married, responded: "Now and forever."

The Rose and Rosow (1972) study analyzed 57,514 initial complaints for divorce, separate maintenance, and annulment in California during the first 6 months of 1968. Divorce rates were highest in the specialties of orthopedic surgery and psychiatry. Small-town doctors had a higher divorce rate than urban doctors. The rate was highest between the ages of 35 and 44. The average divorcing physician was not married until his 30s, lived with his spouse more than 12 years before they were separated, and was over 43 when the initial complaint was filed. The average amount of time spent with patients in a medical specialty was inversely correlated with its divorce rate. Specialists seeing fewer patients, such as pathologists and preventive medicine specialists, tended to have more stable marriages. White male physicians had a lower divorce rate than the general population, but female doctors were at least 40 percent more prone to divorce than men, and black physicians nearly 70 percent more likely to divorce than their white colleagues.

Garvey and Tuason (1979) surveyed 100 randomly selected physicians in the St. Paul (Minnesota) area and received 80 responses that raised questions about a number of common assumptions. The quality of the marriage was not correlated with the educational level of the spouse, nor did it depend on whether the spouse worked outside the home, when in the physician's career the marriage occurred, or the number of hours the physician worked. The marriage was more likely to be good if the husband and wife were rated as extroverted. Garvey and Tuason speculated that physicians and their spouses tend to stay in poor marriages because of such factors as financial security for the spouse and concern about social status in the community.

Stresses on the Medical Marriage

What are the stresses of medical practice that so severely burden the medical marriage? Inescapably, physicians must live with the chronic disparity between the limitations of medicine and their own, the patient's, and society's demands for perfection. They feel a need to be omnipotent, yet are helpless in the face of incurable disease. They are uneasily aware that treatment cannot be provided to everyone in need nor can they possibly know all they need or feel they ought to know. McCue (1982) cited the intense emotional contact with patients, the inability of most patients to express gratitude, and the inadequate preparation for handling difficult patients.

Other pressures come from the need to keep up with new developments in the field (Anwar 1983), paperwork (Krakowski 1982; McCranie et al. 1982), and time demands (Linn et al. 1985; Mawardi 1979; Mechanic 1975). Newer sources of stress are changes in the medical marketplace and the threat of malpractice suits. In a report of a joint American Medical Association–American Psychiatric Association national study of physicians who killed themselves, Sargent (1985) reported that 29 percent of the population of physicians who had successfully completed suicide attempts had been sued for malpractice prior to the attempt.

The recent changes in patterns of practice are another source of stress. Almost all American physicians once worked alone or in small groups in private practice, on a fee-for-service basis. Suddenly a bewildering array of alternatives has arisen: prepaid health maintenance organizations, proprietary hospital corporations, and preferred provider organizations, as well as an equally bewildering variety of reimbursement arrangements. These changes necessarily affect the traditional physician–patient relationship. Physicians increasingly believe that the economics of health care is changing the practice of medicine almost weekly. Patients are choosing their physicians for economic reasons rather than by personal preference; some have physicians chosen for them. Physicians feel overwhelmed, frustrated, and helpless: more like hired technicians and less like health leaders or advocates for the patient.

The expectations of patients and society regarding the physicians' omniscience and invulnerability are tainted with strong ambivalence. The other side of idealization is often contempt. This ambivalence is conveyed in a stanza taken from a 1620 collection of epigrams by John Owen:

God and the doctor we like adore
But only in danger, not before.
The danger is o'er, both alike requited,
God is forgotten and the doctor slighted.

The patient expects the doctor to be available whenever needed, to have time to listen and to empathize with the patient's concerns, to be in a good mood no matter how sleepy or exhausted, to be infallible when it comes to diagnosis and treatment, and to be a paragon of virtuous behavior in the community.

Medical education provides little help in dealing with these stresses. It favors cognitive mastery over interpersonal warmth. Feelings are deemed irrelevant and possibly even a hindrance to "clear thinking." Nonmedical interests are downplayed and discouraged. First-year medical students are commonly advised to turn over all financial and domestic matters to their spouses because the single-minded devotion required of medical training will preclude any attention to household matters such as the checkbook, laundry, cooking, and child rearing. Medical education is also characterized by an active denial of legitimate dependency needs for nurture or support. Personal needs are depreciated and minimized; to the contrary, self-denial, hard work, and suffering are purported to be the *only* route to accomplishment, wisdom, and the respect of one's colleagues.

Unique Features of Medical Marriages

In addition to the problems common to all marriages, medical marriages have special ones related to the demands of practice and the psychological characteristics of physicians. Between the dream and its fulfillment lie a series of unique obstacles to marital fulfillment. These obstacles are the focus of our study.

Physicians hope to find in marriage the nurturance they may see as having been absent or insufficient in childhood or adolescence. The marriage may also provide the prospect of companionship and perhaps a respite from celibacy. For the nonphysician spouse, the marriage offers security and solid comfort as well as a spouse trained in caring for others.

The fulfillment of these partly justifiable hopes is prevented by a shifting barrier of seemingly unavoidable obstacles. Some of these arise from sources that lie beyond the control of the marital pair, in the nature of medicine or in the consequences of couplehood and child rearing. But the most serious stresses arise from within, from the physician's chronic emotional impoverishment, excessive compulsiveness, and single-minded dedication to medicine. Vaillant et al. (1972) found that the occupational hazards of medicine alone do not account for unhappy marriages, substance abuse, and psychological problems in physicians. The presence of such problems is strongly associated with the level of life adjustment before medical school, but only physicians with unstable childhoods were vulnerable to these hazards. In other words, they found that basic personality characteristics, shaped by constitutional-genetic factors and early environment, best predicted marital difficulties and other psychiatric disturbances. We agree; our survey described in Chapter 2 statistically demonstrates this thesis. Chapter 3 is devoted to a more detailed examination of the psychology of the physician.

The plural form in the title of this book is a recognition of the fact that no single type of medical marriage exists. There are numerous variants of physician marriages despite the presence of recurrent, conflictual themes common to many of them. The common denominator in all medical marriages is the psychological makeup of the physician. Physicians tend to be fairly homogenous psychologically, but their spouses are much more diverse. It is perhaps the spouse's individual response to the physician's psychological characteristics that largely determines the presence or absence of conflict in the marriage. The physician's gender also makes a difference; this issue is addressed in Chapters 6 and 7. Eisenberg (1981) noted that while marriage protects men against many sources of dysfunction, for women, marriage acts more like a stressor than a support. According to one survey (Heins et al. 1977b), three-quarters of married female physicians do all of the housework themselves. They are also likely to bear most of the responsibility for child rearing. This may account in part for their very high divorce rate and alarmingly high rate of primary mood disorders—51 percent, according to one survey (Welner et al. 1979).

Long-Term Consequences

For both male and female physicians, marriage introduces two potentially incompatible elements: It is expected to provide emotional sustenance, but it creates a web of obligations to which the physician is less than fully committed. These demands conflict with the commanding responsibilities of medical practice, and medical education has provided no preparation for the conflict. It is virtually impossible to fulfill simultaneously all the roles of a physician and also the roles of a parent and spouse.

Early in the marriage both physician and spouse may view the seeming impossibility of blending personal and professional lives as a temporary problem. The psychology of postponement is crucial; both partners become experts at delayed gratification, a central component in the compulsive makeup of physicians (Coombs 1971; Derdeyn 1978; Ottenberg 1975). The spouses may even admire their husbands or wives for embracing a mature philosophy of work now, play later. Moreover, during medical school or post-graduate training, demanding superiors are a convenient scape-goat. Unfortunately, when training ends, the physician does not slow down as the demands of building a practice become prominent. The realization that things will not change comes slowly and insidiously. Both physician and spouse become perplexed, troubled, angry, and finally resigned to the lack of a satisfactory resolution. The promise of the dream fades.

A languishing death of marital intimacy must certainly affect the quality of the physician's practice—especially the capacity to sustain the outflow of emotional energy required by endless giving to patients. A physician whose marriage is emotionally barren lacks a restoring force that allows him or her to give more to patients. When the marriage helps to meet the physician's own emotional needs, the physician is far better able to meet the demands of needy patients without emotional exhaustion and burn-out.

Conclusion

Partners in a medical marriage are clearly struggling with a fundamentally irreconcilable conflict, a conflict whose essential nature precludes any wholly satisfactory resolution. It is a true dilemma: How can the needs of both the marriage (and later the family) *and* the practice be met? Any solution is at best partial and involves a high-cost trade-off. Strong social forces sharpen each horn of the dilemma, and the generalized institutional indifference to it suggests that a capacity to handle it is believed to be inborn, or God-given, or easily acquired, or unnecessary. Medical schools seldom acknowledge the problem until one partner develops symptoms that require medical or psychiatric intervention. Support groups, often begun by spouses of interns or residents, have been helpful, but they usually operate without official sanction and last only as long as energies and the needs of their founders persist. In short, physicians and their spouses are left to handle the problems themselves, as best they can, without the benefit of teaching based on the wisdom of experience. Our conviction in editing this book has been that the physician's marriage can be either the first casualty of the stress of medical practice *or* the most important resource for coping with that stress. The book reflects our belief that the care and feeding of the medical marriage warrant constructive attention. Studies must address not only the complexities of its inherent dilemmas, but also strategies that can provide help for medical students and their spouses, for specialty training residents and their spouses, and for practicing physicians and their spouses at various stages of professional life. The crisis in medical marriages is a public health problem that deserves more time, energy, and resources than it has received.

The Time of Our Lives: Sources of Conflict in the Medical Marriage

Glen O. Gabbard, M.D.
Roy W. Menninger, M.D.
Lolafaye Coyne, Ph.D.

Studies of medical marriages suggest that often both partners lead what Thoreau called lives of quiet desperation. As noted in Chapter 1, many physicians and spouses report unhappy marriages (Evans 1965; Gerber 1983; Vaillant et al. 1972), but they rarely divorce to seek new partners (Garvey and Tuason 1979; Rose and Rosow 1972). In their elegant prospective study of 47 physicians and 79 controls matched for age, sex, and socioeconomic status, Vaillant et al. (1972) found that 47 percent of the physicians had unhappy marriages as compared to 32 percent of the controls.

In the literature, conflict in medical marriages is usually blamed on the physician's long hours, which leave little time for the family (Elliot 1979; Evans 1965; Gerber 1983; Goldberg 1975; Linn et al. 1985; Mawardi 1979; McCue 1982; Ottenberg 1975; Rhoads 1977; Vincent 1969). But careful studies of physicians find no correlation between long hours of work and the presence of either unhappy marriages or divorces (Garvey and Tuason 1979; Vaillant et al. 1972).

Our study would suggest that the physician's long work hours are often more an effect than a cause of marital problems. Long hours may indicate a characterological compulsiveness (Gabbard

1985; Krakowski 1982; Ottenberg 1975) but they may also serve as a way of avoiding the problems of an unhappy marriage (Evans 1965; Miles et al. 1975; Vaillant et al. 1972; Vincent 1969). Often there is a clash between the character style of the compulsive workaholic physician and the frustrated needs for affection and nurture of the spouse (Evans 1965; Shortt 1979). The physician may avoid open conflict with his or her spouse by prescribing medications or by spending more time at the office (Vaillant et al. 1972). In the traditional marriage of male physician and female nonphysician spouse, tension may arise from the woman's feeling that her identity is contingent on her husband's (Zemon-Gass and Nichols 1975) and from a failure to delineate the roles of each spouse in the marriage (Glick and Borus 1984; Zabarenko et al. 1970).

Blaming lack of time is a rationalization for troubles from other sources. If we physicians are to minimize the suffering of ourselves, our colleagues, and our families, we need a better understanding of marital problems in medical marriages. To this end, we report the results of the following survey.

Method

During the summer of 1985, we surveyed 240 medical couples who participated in the Estes Park workshop. We sent each physician and each spouse a questionnaire. The answers were anonymous and confidentiality was assured. The questionnaires included a 5-point scale measuring marriage gratification and a list of 15 sources of marital conflict. Each respondent was asked to rate these issues on a scale of 0 to 5, according to their importance in his or her marriage. A zero rating indicated that the issue was "not applicable" as a source of conflict in the respondent's marriage; a rating of 1 indicated "of limited importance," 2 "of mild importance," 3 "of moderate importance," 4 "of considerable importance," and 5 "of paramount importance." Each physician and each husband or wife was also asked to rate, on the same 0 to 5 scale, the applicability to his or her partner of 12 frequently heard complaints about spouses.

Results

Of the 240 physician questionnaires, 55.8 percent (134) were returned. Of the 240 spouse questionnaires, 52.1 percent (125) were returned. Of the responding physicians, 93.3 percent (125) were male; of the responding spouses, 97.6 percent (122) were female. In 111 couples both physician and spouse completed a questionnaire. Of these couples, 106 were composed of a male physician and a female nonphysician spouse; two were composed of a female physician and a male nonphysician spouse; and in the remaining three, both partners were physicians. The mean age of the physicians was 44.6; that of the spouses was 42.7. The majority of both physicians and spouses were Caucasian (94.8 and 96.8 percent, respectively). More than 65 percent (88) of the physicians and 67.2 percent (84) of the spouses were Protestant; 12.7 percent (17) of the physicians and 14.4 percent (18) of the spouses were Catholic; 3.7 percent (5) of the physicians and 2.4 percent (3) of the spouses were Jewish. For 90.3 percent (121) of the physicians and 91.2 percent (114) of the spouses, the current marriage was their first. The duration of the marriages ranged from 2 to 55 years, with a mean of 18.8 years. For the spouses, the range was similar, with a mean of 19.2 years. Virtually all the physicians and spouses surveyed were parents; only 2 physicians and 3 spouses in the sample had no children. The modal number of children for both physicians and spouses was 3, with a range of 1 to 7. Although physicians from both rural and metropolitan areas responded to the survey, our sample was skewed toward the rural or small-town practitioner. Some 50.7 percent (68) lived in cities with a population of less than 50,000; only 13.4 percent (18) lived in population centers greater than 500,000. Of the spouses, 84.8 percent (106) had at least a college degree, and 60 percent (75) were employed outside the home. The occupations of the spouses are listed in Table 1.

Table 1. Occupations of Spouses

Occupations	%	N
Homemaker	34.4	43
Profession requiring bachelor's degree	27.2	34
Owner, manager or partner of a small business	11.2	14
Profession requiring advanced degree	7.2	9
Secretary or bookkeeper	7.2	9
Mental health professional	4.8	6
Student	0.8	1
Skilled worker or craftsperson	0.8	1
Owner or executive of large business	0.8	1
Other	0.8	1

The physicians were almost equally divided between primary care practitioners (55.3 percent) and specialists (44.7 percent). Table 2 indicates the breakdown by specialty. Our sample consisted largely of frontline practitioners. Only 5.2 percent (7) worked primarily in an academic setting; 28.4 percent (38) were in solo practice, 24.6 percent (33) in a single specialty group, and 29.1 percent (39) in a multispecialty group. Among the 120 who worked full time, the mean workweek was 56.4 hours.

Mental Health and Marital Satisfaction

Like the group studied by Vaillant et al. (1972), our subjects were relatively healthy psychologically. Only 5 of the physicians and 4 of the spouses had had inpatient psychiatric treatment; 3 physicians and 1 spouse, alcoholism treatment; 3 physicians and no spouse, drug abuse treatment; and 33 physicians and 26 spouses, outpatient psychiatric treatment.

Nevertheless, 47 percent (63) of the physicians and 48 percent (60) of the spouses had sought marital counseling. These percent-

Table 2. Medical Specialties of Physician Group Specialty

Medical Specialty	%	N
Family or general practice	43.3	58
Adult or child psychiatry	14.9	20
Internal medicine	7.5	10
Pediatrics	4.5	6
General surgery	3.7	5
Emergency medicine	3.0	4
Obstetrics and gynecology	3.0	4
Ophthalmology	2.2	3
Anesthesiology	1.5	2
Cardiology	1.5	2
Oncology	1.5	2
Pathology	1.5	2
Orthopedic surgery	1.5	2
Dermatology	0.8	1
Gastroenterology	0.8	1
Nuclear medicine	0.8	1
Ear, nose, and throat	0.8	1
Clinical pharmacology	0.8	1
Diagnostic radiology	0.8	1
Therapeutic radiology	0.8	1
Head and neck surgery	0.8	1
Thoracic surgery	0.8	1
Urology	0.8	1
Other	3.0	4

Table 3. Rating of Marriage Gratification by Physicians and Their
Spouses

Rating of Marriage Gratification	Physicians		Spouses	
	%	N	%	N
1—Extremely gratifying	32.8	44	28.8	36
2—Moderately gratifying	45.5	61	40.8	51
3—Mixed	11.2	15	19.2	24
4—Moderately nongratifying	8.2	11	4.8	6
5—Extremely nongratifying	.75	1	4.8	6

ages are virtually identical to the incidence of unhappy marriages
in Vaillant et al.'s (1972) study. Another 20.9 percent (28) of the
physicians and 16.9 percent (21) of the spouses in our sample had
seriously considered marital counseling. Thus 68 percent of the
physicians and 65 percent of the spouses had either sought or
considered marital counseling. This number makes their answers
to questions on marital gratification rather puzzling. As Table 3
shows, most said their marriages were either extremely gratifying
or moderately gratifying. How are we to understand this apparent
discrepancy?

One explanation is that the respondents have happy marriages
because of counseling. However, analysis of the data suggests that
this is not so. Physicians who never considered marital counseling
found their marriages more gratifying ($M = 1.48$) than did those
who sought marital counseling ($M = 2.31$) or those who considered
marital counseling ($M = 2.09$) ($p < .01$ in both comparisons).*
Similar differences were found among spouses.

Another possibility is that couples with serious problems may
call their marriages moderately or extremely gratifying simply
because of low expectations or a need to project an image of har-
mony. Low expectations are suggested by the fact that 48 respondents, many of whom had rated their marriages as gratifying,
appended written comments describing a variety of marital difficulties. Separation or divorce had been considered by 29.1 percent (39) of the physicians and 38.4 percent (48) of the spouses.

Our findings call to mind another study that was completed
20 years ago (Owens 1966). Questionnaires were mailed to 403
physicians and 323 physicians' wives in that survey. Only 5 percent of the wives and 4 percent of the physicians admitted being
very dissatisfied with their spouses. However, nearly a quarter of

---

*Following a significant overall F test, we used the Newman-Keuls test for com-
parison of pairs of means.

the sample had sought help for marital or family problems. That finding may only have reflected the ready access of physicians to mental health professionals. But Coombs (1971) offered an interpretation that agrees with ours: "Doctors and their wives, in order to maintain a good public image, tend to give socially approved rather than strictly accurate replies to inquiries about their marital success" (p. 134).

The physicians in our sample lived up to the stereotype that portrays them as too busy and too tired for sex. The mean frequency of sexual relations was 1.6 times a week, with a range from 0 (10.5 percent of the sample) to 6 (0.8 percent). The modal frequency of sexual relations was once a week, reported by 27.6 percent. This low frequency was not due to a disproportionate number of older men. For physicians age 42 or older, the mean frequency of sexual relations per week was 1.3; for those under 42, the frequency was 1.8 per week. The difference was not statistically significant.

Perceptions of Sources of Conflict

Table 4 shows how physicians and spouses ranked sources of marital conflict on the 0 to 5 scale described earlier. Physicians and spouses rank the sources of conflict fairly similarly; for example, "lack of time for fun, family, and self" ranks first on both lists. But there are two major discrepancies. First, physicians see "amount of time away from home at work" as a much more important source of conflict than spouses do. Second, spouses consider "lack of intimacy" a much more serious problem than physicians do.

Since these data come from all responding physicians and spouses as a group, it is hard to tell without further analysis whether differing perceptions of problems exist within each marriage. We therefore took a closer statistical look at the 111 married couples who sent in completed questionnaires.

Table 5 demonstrates that individual husband and wife pairs tend to rate the importance of items *differently* rather than agreeing on their sources of conflict. The five areas of greatest disagreement, in order from the most to the least discrepant, are: (1) "tension in the family home," (2) "quality of sexual relations," (3) "finances," (4) "lack of intimacy," and (5) "religious differences."

We also asked physicians and spouses to rate on a 0 to 5 scale the importance of various problems that they perceived in their

Table 4. Sources of Conflict Cited by Physicians and Their Spouses

Source of Conflict	Rank Order of Physicians' Ratings	Rank Order of Spouses' Ratings
Lack of time for fun, family, and self	1	1
Amount of time away from home at work	2	8
Frequency of sexual relations	3	4
Finances	4	5
Money management	5	3
Tension in the family home	6	7
Lack of intimacy	7	2
Lack of shared responsibilities for children and for work around the house	8	6
Philosophy of child rearing	9	9
Quality of sexual relations	10	10
In-laws	11	11
Family size	12	15
Jealousy	12	13
Religious differences	14	14
Taboo subjects	15	12

Table 5. Pearson Product-Moment Correlations Between Individual Physicians' and Spouses' Ratings of the Sources of Marital Conflict

Source of Conflict	r^*	df	p
Lack of time for fun, family, and self	.417	83	.001
Amount of time away from home at work	.441	86	.001
Frequency of sexual relations	.481	82	.001
Finances	.291	83	.01
Money management	.458	82	.001
Tension in the family home	.279	85	.01
Lack of intimacy	.296	80	.01
Lack of shared responsibilities for children and for work around the house	.438	81	.001
Philosophy of child rearing	.445	84	.001
Quality of sexual relations	.287	81	.01
In-laws	.397	84	.001
Family size	.533	85	.001
Jealousy	.424	82	.001
Religious differences	.341	81	.01
Taboo subjects	.466	84	.001

*If this analysis is viewed as similar to a reliability test, one can readily see that on *no* item among the entire list of 15 do husband and wife approach the .7 or .8 figures that are considered acceptable levels of reliability, indicating about 50 percent shared variance.

marital partners. Table 6 shows the answers. A cursory glance reveals major discrepancies. The primary concern of physicians is that their spouses are not interested in sex; the primary complaint of the spouses is that their physician spouses will not talk to them. Physicians also rank "doesn't listen to me" high as a complaint; the data suggest that one reason physicians do not talk to their spouses as much as their spouses would like is that they do not expect their spouses to listen.

Again we checked for discrepancies within each marriage. As Table 7 suggests, the responses here are even more discrepant than the responses to questions about sources of conflict in the relationship. Two items here are actually negatively correlated. "Expects too much from me sexually," for example, was given a 4 or 5 rating by 12 spouses; no physicians rated it either 4 or 5. "Is not interested in sexual activity" was rated 1 (not a problem) by 60 spouses but only by 26 physicians. Other problems most discrepantly perceived are, in descending order: (*1*) "complains too much," (*2*) "nags me too much about my lack of time at home," (*3*) "doesn't listen to me," and (*4*) "pays more attention to other members of the opposite sex than to me."

Tension, Time, and Absence from Home

To clarify whether the number of hours spent at work was truly the major source of tension in medical marriages, we com-

Table 6. Importance of Problems Perceived in Marital Partner

Problem Perceived in Marital Partner	Physician Perception of Spouse	Spouse Perception of Physician
Is not interested in sexual activity	1	9
Doesn't empathize with my role and position	2	4
Doesn't listen to me	3	3
Expects too much work around the house from me	4	8
Complains too much	5	7
Doesn't provide enough emotional support for me	6	2
Nags me too much about my lack of time at home	7	10
Doesn't talk to me enough	8	1
Doesn't respect me enough	9	5
Expects too much from me sexually	10	6
Jealousy	11	11
Pays more attention to other members of the opposite sex than to me	12	12

Note. Data represent mean ratings in rank order.

Table 7. Pearson Product-Moment Correlations Between
Physicians' and Spouses' Views of Problems in the
Marital Partner

Problem Perceived in Marital Partner	r	df	p
Is not interested in sexual activity	$-.140$	104	NS
Doesn't empathize with my role and position	.258	104	.01
Doesn't listen to me	.110	104	NS
Expects too much work around the house from me	.255	104	.05
Complains too much	.032	104	NS
Doesn't provide enough emotional support for me	.377	104	.001
Nags me too much about my lack of time at home	.038	104	NS
Doesn't talk to me enough	.240	103	.05
Doesn't respect me enough	.406	103	.001
Expects too much from me sexually	$-.205$	104	.05
Jealousy	.264	104	.01
Pays more attention to other members of the opposite sex than to me	.138	104	NS

pared physicians who worked more than 60 hours per week with
those who worked between 40 and 50 hours per week.*

Physicians in the former group rated "lack of time for fun,
family, and self" higher as a source of tension than those who
worked fewer hours ($M = 3.61$ vs $M = 2.96, p < .02$), but they did
not say their marriages were less happy, and their spouses agreed.
In fact, the physicians who worked longer hours had sexual relations more often (1.7 vs 1.3 times a week), although the difference
was not statistically significant.

We also compared primary care practitioners and specialists.
Primary care practitioners regarded their marriages as significantly *more* gratifying than did specialists ($M = 1.78$ vs $M = 2.20$,
$p < .01$). Again, spouses agreed ($M = 1.92$ vs $M - 2.33, p < .05$).
Solo and group practitioners did not differ in level of marital
happiness, nor did their spouses. Earlier studies had suggested
greater marital unhappiness and divorce among rural physicians
(Rose and Rosow 1972), but we found no significant urban-rural
differences.

Finally, we compared the 43 physicians who had never considered or sought marital counseling with the 91 who had. We
found that the physicians who sought marital counseling averaged
30.5 minutes per day talking with their spouses; those who considered marital counseling averaged 38.8 minutes per day; and

*Univariate independent group *t* tests were used. Because of varying numbers,
multivariate analyses were not possible. To guard against chance results, only consistent patterns of findings are reported here.

those who neither considered nor sought marital counseling averaged 57.3 minutes per day ($p < .001$). Among the spouses, those who sought marital counseling averaged 41.6 minutes of talking per day; those who considered marital counseling averaged 42.7 minutes per day; and those who neither considered nor sought marital counseling averaged 61 minutes per day ($p < .05$). Cause and effect cannot be established here, but the findings are certainly consistent with the conclusion that couples who communicate more have less need for marital counseling. It is worth noting that the frequency of sexual relations did not differ significantly among these three groups.

Discussion

Our findings must be cautiously interpreted. They cannot be readily generalized to two-physician marriages or to those involving only a female physician. A second limitation is that our sample was self-selected; only couples who came to a seminar for physicians and their families participated. However, our workshop has not attracted mostly disturbed couples in search of marital therapy. On the contrary, our data suggest that participants tend to be psychologically healthy. The workshop is described as a continuing medical education (CME) seminar, not as treatment or therapy. Many participants simply enjoy the opportunity to combine an educational experience for CME credits with a family vacation in a beautiful setting. Nevertheless, physicians and spouses who are open to reviewing their relationship may be quite different from those who are not. The low incidence of impairment in our sample may reflect this difference.

We are not claiming that these sources of conflict occur only in the marriages of physicians. We had no control group of other professionals. But the high proportion of poor medical marriages has already been demonstrated by a sophisticated prospective study with controls (Vaillant et al. 1972). Our goal was to examine a group of physician marriages in more detail to gain a better understanding of the sources of that discord. A unique feature of our study is the examination of a large sample of *both* physicians and spouses in which the physician is a nonacademic, frontline practitioner. Previous studies have concentrated on academic settings, and they have focused on either physicians or spouses, but not on both.

Within the limitations of our data, we can conclude that lack of time due to the demands of practice seems to be a complaint that serves the function of externalizing the conflicts *in* the marriage onto factors *outside* the marriage, but it is not the primary cause of marital dysfunction. Our study suggests that differing needs for intimacy, differing perceptions of problems in the marital relationship, and differing communication styles are the chief sources of conflict in medical marriages.

Discrepancies in communication styles may be fundamental. The spouses prefer verbal communication and are disappointed that their physician spouses do not share this preference. Physicians tend to be compulsive and emotionally inexpressive (Gabbard 1985; Krakowski 1982); this bent, augmented by medical training and practice, leads them to suppress and deny their feelings and to utilize nonverbal actions to express emotion. Perhaps sexual activity is one of the few ways physicians have to express affection to their spouses. In contrast, the physicians' primary complaint is their spouses' lack of sexual interest, but this too may express a communication problem. When the physician wishes to make love, the spouse often wants to talk. In the resulting emotional "dialogue of the deaf," efforts to communicate fail, leaving each partner with unmet emotional needs and the feeling that he or she is misunderstood. Eventually such discrepancies lead to chronic marital dissatisfaction.

Our finding of an association between marital happiness and the time a couple spends talking suggests several hypotheses for testing. It is tempting to assume a cause-and-effect relationship, but the association may simply reflect similarities or differences in communication styles. In other words, in marriages rated happier, both partners may be comfortable with verbal expression of feelings. Another possible interpretation is that dissatisfied couples talk less because they see the sources or consequences of conflict differently. Repeated efforts to clarify and resolve tensions may only lead to further disagreements and finally hostile stalemate.

Another finding that deserves comment is the greater marital happiness of primary care practitioners as compared to specialists. Physicians drawn to a specialist career may be less comfortable with the long-term emotional relationships that develop between primary care practitioners and their patients. Because they treat isolated organ systems, specialists can establish greater emotional distance from the patient and can more readily rely on such defenses as isolation and displacement. This may carry over into the marriage and contribute to a lower level of gratification.

The patterns of discrepancy between physicians and spouses that we have demonstrated should be compared with those of other populations of physicians and their spouses to deepen our understanding of the dynamics of medical marriages. Time may indeed be our ultimate master, but to understand more fully the insidious desperation that sometimes seeps into our lives, we must look first at ourselves and our most intimate relationships.

The Psychology of the Physician

Glen O. Gabbard, M.D.
Roy W. Menninger, M.D.

It is just as unbearable to be God as it is to remain an utter slave.
—Otto Rank, *Beyond Psychology*, 1941

One spring morning not long ago, Dr. A., a general surgeon in a Western state, started driving from his home to a small town where he held a clinic once a week. His wife had been depressed that day, and she made it clear that she was upset about his going out of town. He thought about that as he departed, and 10 miles past the city limits he turned around to come back. All the way home he ruminated about whether he was shirking his responsibility by not attending the surgical clinic. A general practitioner in the town where the clinic was located became annoyed at Dr. A. for not showing up, because he had a patient waiting who needed emergency surgery. Fortunately another surgeon was able to perform the operation. Nevertheless, Dr. A. felt guilty about disregarding his obligation to that patient.

Five months later, the case was presented by the operating surgeon at a conference at the hospital with which Dr. A. was affiliated. The presentation reawakened his guilt. When he told his wife about it, she took his remarks as a personal attack and an insinuation that he was sorry he had returned home. Three nights later she committed suicide. From then on, Dr. A. was haunted relentlessly by even more intense guilt.

Although this tragic ending is unusual, the vast majority of physicians have similar struggles, which reflect certain common personality traits. They are conscientious about attending to the needs of both their practices and their families. They make futile efforts to please everyone that leave them with the feeling that they have pleased no one. They have an exaggerated sense of responsibility that makes them feel guilty about things beyond their control. Their unrelenting perfectionism and chronic self-doubt produce a profound sense that they are never doing enough. Although in reality his wife's suicide was the result of long-term emotional disturbance, including a severe chronic depression, Dr. A.'s feelings resonate with the guilt we all feel for choosing practice over family—time and time again. Shortly after the suicide, Dr. A. was attending a Jewish service on Yom Kippur, the Day of Atonement, when the following words from one of the readings leapt off the page at him: "Some have made idols of professional advancement, social status, and material reward. Some, while pretending to love humanity, have withheld from their own people the love they deserve." Virtually every physician experiences a little self-recognition in those words.

It is tempting to blame conflict in the physician's marriage on external factors, such as the stress of practice and the way of life society imposes on the physician. But physicians' practices and life-styles reflect their psychology. As the study described in Chapter 2 suggests, the time demands of a busy medical practice are rarely the real cause of marital problems. These demands more often serve as rationalizations to justify preserving the emotional distance that physicians are characterologically prone to create in their personal relationships. To understand the recurrent patterns of conflict in medical marriages, one must first understand the psychological makeup of the typical physician.

Childhood Origins

The adult personality of the physician results from a defensive style adopted in early childhood to deal with what is perceived as parental failure to provide adequate emotional nurturance. This defensive style colors all subsequent relationships with patients, colleagues, and spouses. Vaillant et al. (1972) noted that physicians with primary responsibility for patient care were more likely to have had emotionally impoverished childhoods than a control group of nonphysicians. According to Vaillant and his colleagues, frontline practitioners may be using medicine as a way of giving to patients the care and attention they feel they lacked as children.

In our clinical and educational work, we have repeatedly confirmed this hypothesis.

This is not to say that the parents of future physicians really
were emotionally distant; the important point is that the physician sees them that way. Future physicians possibly require more
parental encouragement and reassurance than the ordinary child
if they are to feel loved and valued. The parents are not villains;
both child and parent contribute to the difficulty.

The child has strong unfulfilled dependent yearnings and feels
angry at the parents for not being more emotionally available.
Because both the rage and the dependent wishes are uncomfortable, the child defends against them by reaction formation: giving
to others as a way of denying anger and neediness. Vaillant et al.
(1972) found this to be one of the chief defense mechanisms that
differentiated physicians from controls in their study. Self-denial
reassures physicians that their dependency needs are well under
control. By devoting their lives to helping others, they attempt to
conquer their guilt for feeling angry at their parents (Gerber 1983;
Rhoads 1977). The typical physician wages a constant struggle to
keep aggressive impulses under control and make sure they are
not expressed through misdiagnosis, sloppy treatment, or neglect
of duties. This anxiety about aggression is what distinguishes the
workaholic physician from the workaholic lawyer or business-
person. As Karl Menninger (1957) noted, the practice of medicine
affords "a unique opportunity to conceal conscious or unconscious
sadism" (p. 101).

The need to control others is also an important component of
the doctor's personality. This involves not only an effort to control
aggression arising from unconscious wishes for revenge against
emotionally distant parents, but also a wish to control the sources
of love and support in the environment. Unconsciously, physicians
expect that their dedicated, selfless care will make others so grateful that they will respond with emotional support. The child felt
essentially unloved; the adult feels a need to make heroic efforts
to prove his or her value and receive the longed-for admiration.

Yet strangely, physicians are uncomfortable when patients or
family members express their gratitude in a loving way. The long-
delayed reward of appreciation and admiration does not provide
the hoped-for gratification because the wish for love has been
transmuted into a need for generalized esteem. The respect of
colleagues, patients, and the community replaces the original desire for an intimate relationship with a loving parent. Physicians'

spouses commonly complain that their husbands or wives worry more about what their colleagues think than about what their families think. Spousal expressions of warmth and tenderness are met with an uncomfortable, aloof response. As one doctor's wife put it, "Sometimes when I hug him, I feel like no one's there, and it scares me."

This transmutation of parental love into an abstraction is a natural outgrowth of the physician's fears about emotional intimacy. As our survey demonstrated, physicians appear to have much less need for intimacy than their spouses. Elliot (1979) made a similar observation in her study of 38 British hospital doctors and their wives:

> The loneliness that most hospital doctors' wives experienced as resulting from the curtailment of shared home leisure is experienced by only 16 percent of hospital doctors. Their accounts suggest that the social relationships of work provide them with expressive satisfactions—that they do not have the same need for connubial companionship that their wives have. (p. 60)

Both dependent yearnings and anxiety about aggression make physicians wary of intimacy. They fear being overwhelmed by powerful wishes to be taken care of, and they also fear that destructive aggression will emerge. Courting the world's esteem allows physicians to feel good about themselves without the threat of intimacy.

Medical practice provides the male physician with the means for achieving a modest level of intimacy with his patients in a controlled way—satisfying but not so close as to be difficult or threatening: his businesslike manner, his diagnostic procedures, the presence of office personnel, and most of all, the need for close attention to the diagnostic and therapeutic tasks. With his spouse and family, on the other hand, the demands for intimacy are equally great but the absence of the structure provided by the practice forces the physician to resort to other distancing techniques: indifference, avoidance, preoccupation with "important matters" or life-threatening illnesses, and ultimately, the unchallengeable defense of flight from home into the practice.

Our survey findings also suggest that physicians often disconnect sexual relations from emotional intimacy. The amount of sexual activity in these marriages was not correlated with the physician's workload or the amount of time the couple spent talking each day. The spouses, most of whom were women, wanted more intimacy but were not particularly concerned about the frequency or quality of their sexual relations. Their husbands did not see lack of intimacy as a problem but tended to think their wives were not sexually responsive enough. Physicians' sexual lives are often conducted in the same cool, detached, compulsive style that characterizes their professional practice, and their wives may feel a disappointing lack of emotional closeness during lovemaking. In Chapter 8 Domeena Renshaw provides some illuminating illustrations of this disconnection between sexuality and intimacy in the everyday life of physician couples.

Perfectionism

Physicians are often said to be narcissistic. No doubt some of them act in a way that has inspired the caricature of the vain, self-aggrandizing prima donna who assigns an intern the job of opening doors. But that is certainly not typical. The narcissism of most physicians is subtler. Rothstein (1980) removed the pejorative connotations from the term *narcissism* by defining it as a pursuit of perfection that is in itself neither healthy nor pathological. Narcissistic psychopathology develops only when this pursuit is integrated by a pathological ego rather than a healthy one. Feelings of helplessness and vulnerability may produce strivings for perfection in oneself, or they may create the wish to live in the shadow of another person who is viewed as perfect. Perfectionism is so common in physicians that such prior feelings of helplessness and vulnerability must be common motivators in the choice of a medical career.

According to Rothstein (1980), a child's pursuit of perfection may take the form of idealizing the parent. This image of a perfect parent is eventually internalized as a presence that is felt to be part of oneself. The child then gains self-esteem by performing successfully for the internal parent. Thus physicians may feel that they can capture the approval of the perfect parent and the accompanying blissful feelings if they can only achieve perfection.

In a classic paper, Rhoads (1977) observed that workaholics often need to be loved by everyone. The physicians' long hours may be an effort to achieve that goal, and transcending any hint of aggression is an integral part of it. A person who is slavishly, selflessly devoted to the care of patients is above reproach. How could anyone accuse such a saintly martyr of being destructive, mean, selfish, or lazy? Moreover, the physician's fantasy of becoming perfectly competent is a way of fending off a continuing sense of inadequacy. Perfection in one's practice, the physician unconsciously believes, will produce a perfect transcendent state of love.

A parent's soothing, adoring attention is the child's first source of self-esteem. Eventually the physician obtains a similar emotional response by living up to the standards of an internalized version of the parent: in psychoanalytic terms, an aspect of the superego. Professors or other professional role models may become endowed with the qualities of this internalized parent. The medical student or resident feels that working 36 hours straight without sleep is worth the effort if it pleases the attending physician. Spouses rarely take on so much importance; their esteem and praise are less crucial. The demands of the internalized parent also explain why praise, admiration, and love never seem adequate to satisfy the physician's longings. This parent who has become part of the self can no more be satisfied than the physician's real parents seemed to have been. The result is self-doubt, a key characteristic that distinguished physicians from controls in Vaillant et al.'s (1972) study. No matter how many diplomas grace their office walls, no matter how many operations they have successfully performed, no matter how great the respect of their colleagues, many physicians secretly lack self-confidence. The aura of power and authority with which they surround themselves is often a defensive posture designed to ward off daily reminders of fallibility—treatment failures, dissatisfied patients, continued pain and suffering.

Nothing exposes the physician's fragile self-esteem so clearly as a malpractice suit. It can penetrate the veneer of self-confidence and reveal the underlying anxiety about self-worth and competence. When sued, even the most competent and respected physicians will often become convinced that they have lost all respect in the eyes of the community and colleagues.

Many physicians find that the void cannot be filled. When they are praised or loved, they mistrust the admiration or attention. It is one more aspect of the impossible dream; physicians strive endlessly to receive something that they always experience as unattainable or at best inadequate.

This helps us to understand the apparent masochism of physicians. Vaillant et al. (1972) noted that they do not strive primarily for pleasure or instinctual gratification. Rather, their pleasure and sense of self-esteem come in the form of *relief* from the relentless and tormenting demands of the internalized parent. Combined with the wish to control aggression and the sources of love, this contributes to the need for mastery and perfection.

Compulsiveness in the Normal Physician

Most of the characteristics described above are compulsive personality traits. In a prominent Midwestern medical school, a professor of internal medicine grandly stated to a group of eager first-year medical students in a course on physical diagnosis: "The most important quality of a physician is compulsiveness." His audience, no doubt, was compulsively writing down every word, underlining every important phrase, and preparing to commit the entire text to memory. Although other medical educators might challenge the professor's view of its importance, there is no doubt that compulsiveness is the hallmark of the physician's personality (Gabbard 1985; Krell and Miles 1976; Rhoads 1977; Waring 1974). In a poll of 100 randomly selected physicians, Krakowski (1982) found that all declared themselves to be "compulsive personalities." Eighty percent satisfied three of the five criteria given for this diagnosis in the current psychiatric diagnostic manual, and 20 percent satisfied four of the five criteria. These are: (*1*) restricted ability to express warm and tender emotions, (*2*) perfectionism, (*3*) insistence that others submit to one's way of doing things, (*4*) excessive devotion to work and productivity to the exclusion of pleasure and interpersonal relationships, and (*5*) indecisiveness. All physicians do not have compulsive personality disorders; but compulsive *traits* are present in most people who turn to medicine as a profession. The pursuit of perfection, then, may be viewed as one of several compulsive traits found in most physicians.

Why do physicians have these traits? They are not associated simply with high professional positions; attorneys, for example, are much less compulsive (Krakowski 1984). Although a certain type of personality is undoubtedly drawn to the profession of medicine, medical education itself enhances compulsiveness. The premedical curriculum, medical school, and the stresses of residency foster the development of defense mechanisms typical of compulsive personalities (Keniston 1967; Nadelson and Notman 1979).

What are the consequences for the physician? As Bittker (1976) noted, many of the character traits that contribute to success in medical practice create a risk of depression when they are exaggerated or carried to an extreme. Sargent (1986) found that the same personality traits that predispose a person to a medical career may also increase vulnerability to suicide.

Many physicians can be characterized by a particular compulsive triad of doubt, guilt feelings, and an exaggerated sense of responsibility (Gabbard 1985) that has both adaptive and maladaptive aspects. A healthy sense of doubt makes for diagnostic rigor, leading the physician to check and double-check laboratory data and physical findings for discrepancies and for minute changes that might be significant. Thoroughness is essential in medicine. We would all probably prefer a compulsive physician if we were seriously ill. This is the paradox: Compulsiveness is socially valuable, but personally expensive. Society's meat is the physician's poison.

But doubt can also become tormenting for physicians. They may be obsessed with the notion that something important has been missed, and the patient will deteriorate. Self-doubt and indecisiveness may even interfere with the physician's professional functioning.

> A case in point is Dr. B., a 39-year-old neurologist. Although she was respected as a dedicated and serious-minded clinician, the residents and medical students on her service regularly registered complaints about her to the department chairperson. When Dr. B. made rounds, she would take hours to examine a handful of patients. In performing a neurological examination, she often checked the patient's foot 20 or 30 times to be absolutely certain that a Babinski reflex was absent. Medical students and residents became bored and resentful as they stood and watched her perform this obsessive examination ritual with patient after patient, while their paperwork and other responsibilities mounted. She also showed what they saw as disrespect for their abilities by doubting any findings they presented and insisting on confirming them herself. Ultimately Dr. B.'s indecisiveness led her to change specialties. With the support of her department chair, she entered a pathology residency, where she could exercise her obsessional doubt in relative isolation, with less immediate impact on colleagues and trainees.

Guilt feelings, the second component of the compulsive triad, may also cause considerable misery. If a patient dies, for example, the physician is too likely to feel that he or she is personally to blame. This proneness to guilt is intimately connected with the third element of the triad, an exaggerated sense of responsibility. Certainly physicians should have a strong sense of responsibility; it is a source of professional pride and ethical conduct. However, when taken to an extreme, this trait may verge on fantasized omnipotence. Obviously the physician is not always to blame when a patient dies. The patient's health habits may have been poor; an unexpected drug reaction may have occurred; or fate, the natural course of events, may be the culprit. Nevertheless, physicians are likely to recall vividly and uneasily postmortem conferences in which an apparently self-assured and condescending pathologist claimed to be able to point out exactly where the attending physician had erred and how the patient's death could have been prevented.

> Dr. C., a 52-year-old family practitioner, agonized for years over having "killed" one of his patients 17 years before. He had given a young man penicillin for a bacterial pharyngitis; the patient went into anaphylactic shock before his eyes and died. For many years the physician went over that office visit in his mind. He had to reassure himself repeatedly that the patient had denied any allergy to penicillin. He consulted colleagues and had lengthy discussions with the pathologist who performed the autopsy. They all told him that he was not responsible: "It could have happened to anyone." He has spent many hours poring over articles on anaphylactic shock and its treatment, and still sometimes lies awake at night obsessively reviewing the details of that event.

Such guilt feelings are not just the result of a failure of the physician's defenses against aggressive feelings. They are also a response to a sense of inadequacy and helplessness. One reason for choosing medicine as a profession may be a need to defend against the horrible existential dread associated with feelings of impotence in the face of one's own death (Kasper 1959; Krakowski 1971). In other words, physicians may pursue medicine to prevent themselves from feeling helpless as well as to prevent themselves from hurting others. They often have an unconscious feeling of omnipotence in the form of exaggerated expectations—feelings integrally related to the narcissistic pursuit of perfection. Any physician who harbors unconscious or conscious fantasies about outwrestling the Angel of Death will be prone to take the blame when death wins the match. Medicine is ultimately only palliative; it is another grand paradox that people who are so vulnerable to feelings of helplessness choose a profession that repeatedly reminds them of their impotence in the face of disease and death.

All these concerns may lead physicians to work exceedingly long hours in an effort to clear their consciences (Rhoads 1977). Overwork is also caused by the need to be needed. Just as actors need the applause of an audience for emotional survival, so physicians need to be valued and needed by their patients. Children who grow up to be doctors tend to be uncertain about their value. Terman's (1954) study of 800 gifted men demonstrated that, as a group, physicians tend to feel inferior. This insecurity drives them to seek approval through more responsibility, more work, and more self-denial.

One obvious consequence is a severe restriction of leisure time. In Krakowski's (1982) sample of 100 physicians, only 16 read or watched television for pleasure or attended theater or concerts. Only 10 regularly took time off to relax, and a mere 11 took vacations exclusively for vacation's sake. Their usual reaction to stress was to *increase* their professional activity rather than take time off. What leisure physicians do take is guilt-ridden. They may feel tempted to jog or swim, or develop a hobby, but they often feel guilty about taking time away from families. As one young general practitioner put it, "Time for work comes first; time for family is a distant second; and time for self is an even more distant third."

> Unstructured time often makes busy physicians anxious. Dr. D., a 38-year-old family practitioner in a group practice, looked forward to a rare weekend with no call for his services. Anxiously seeking guidelines, he sat down and made a list of things he had to do during the weekend. There was a growing stack of journals to read; the grass had to be cut; the screen door needed repair; the air conditioner in the car was malfunctioning. The list rapidly grew. By Sunday evening he felt thoroughly frustrated because he had not accomplished all he had set out to do. He had not only robbed himself of free time but had once again avoided meaningful interaction with his family and had intensified his own internal distress.

> A married couple, both busy pediatricians, decided to get away for a week's vacation in the Bahamas. The first morning on the island was quite disconcerting, because they had no schedule to follow. Their response was to begin scheduling activities to structure the week. Every time they walked along the beach, they experienced vague guilt feelings about not "doing something."

Throughout the week they had to remind themselves repeatedly that doing nothing was a legitimate way to spend a vacation. Each of them had to give permission to the other to have a good time without feeling guilty, and even then, they were only partially successful.

This guilt about leisure time is so great that often physicians can justify even swimming or jogging only by persuading themselves that it is for someone else's good; for example, jogging will prevent a heart attack that might leave the family without financial support.

Guilt for having free time may take many forms.

Dr. E., a young cardiologist, ruminated for several months about taking a day off in the middle of the week to spend with his wife. She finally convinced him to take the time so that they could shop for a new sofa together. The physician woke up on his day off with a sense of dread. He felt that it was sneaky and dishonest to stay away from work; his colleagues must be grumbling about his absence. Before he could get out of the door, he was struck with a migraine headache that forced him to go to bed for the rest of the day.

This dramatic example of somatization is not unusual. The physician was punishing himself for the sin of staying home from work. Punishments are built into the physician's life-style as though they are required for the maintenance of equilibrium. Even the dutiful compulsive reading of journals is a form of punishment for some physicians, designed to ameliorate anxiety about never being able to keep up with all they should know. Legal pressures make this process even more guilt-ridden and anxiety-provoking. As we point out at length in Chapter 4, the threat of malpractice suits has seriously eroded the traditional doctor–patient relationship and greatly increased self-doubt and guilt.

Physicians seem to believe that any effort on behalf of themselves is selfish. As Gerber (1983) noted, they equate selfishness with weakness and selflessness with strength. Asserting their own needs would be a violation of the contract implicitly made many years ago with their parents: self-sacrifice guarantees love, while self-assertion alienates one from fundamental sources of nurturance. Because of this trouble in distinguishing healthy self-interest from selfishness, physicians tend to deny their human limitations and human weaknesses while mounting a grand campaign against death and disease, which often leads to self-neglect and self-destructive overwork.

Impact on the Marriage

Patients do not complain about compulsiveness in physicians, and as we have seen, neither do the physicians themselves. Spouses do complain. When a physician will not drive home at the end of the day until the three children with fevers waiting in the office have been seen, hospital rounds have been made, and paperwork completed, the family suffers the consequences. The physician must deal with their disappointment as well as his or her own guilt. More and more physicians are shunning solo practice for the shared coverage arrangement of a group, but the same difficulties persist. Many find it hard to turn over a patient to a colleague at 5 or 6 p.m., when their office hours are supposed to end.

> Dr. F., a 41-year-old family practitioner, was getting ready to leave his office at 6 p.m. to rush home and have supper before attending his son's final high school basketball game. The hospital called to tell him that one of his obstetric patients had arrived in labor and was near delivery. He knew that one of the partners in his group practice was covering obstetrics that night, but he felt compelled to run by the hospital to check her before going home. He decided to stay through the delivery and missed his son's game. After the delivery he sat in the locker room and wept. Why had he not just handed the case over to his partner? He was not even emotionally attached to this patient. His exaggerated sense of responsibility had conquered; he and he alone had to deliver the baby.

This picture is all too familiar to most of us. As we all know, the decision usually goes in favor of the patient rather than the family. The physician is certain of winning the respect of colleagues by making rounds in the evening, and the spouse cannot complain without feeling guilty. After all, the physician husband or wife has been dealing with life and death issues all day. Any concern about the house, the children, or the concert they were supposed to attend may seem trivial by comparison. If the spouse is forgiving and understanding, the physician's guilt increases. If the spouse is critical, the physician may want to stay at the office even later the next time. Often the spouse compromises by swallowing resentment and retreating into silence.

This familiar conflict illustrates how time away from home takes center stage in the theater of marital discord. Among the 200 medical couples that Goldberg (1975) saw in marital therapy, this was first among the spouses' complaints. Similarly, in our survey discussed in Chapter 2, both partners saw the physician's lack of time as the main source of tension in the marriage. The demands of practice are a convenient rationalization. Physicians work long hours to deny dependency; to eradicate any trace of aggression or destructiveness that they fear others may suspect; to win the unconditional love and approval of colleagues, patients, and community; to maintain complete control; and to conquer the terror of death. It is not the demands of practice but the physician's compulsive character that wreaks havoc in the marriage. Our survey suggests that differing intimacy needs, communication styles, and perceptions lie at the root of conflict in medical marriages; all of them are related to the physician's extraordinary compulsiveness.

Dr. G., a 34-year-old chief resident in pediatrics, was dedicated to her patients and trainees. She said to herself that she did not like the long hours but wanted to set a good example for junior residents and medical students under her supervision. Her husband became impatient and told her bluntly that she had her priorities wrong. Dr. G. would treat patients who showed up at 5 or 6 p.m. after being sick all day; her husband told her to send them to the emergency room instead. She also allowed patients to call at all hours with trivial complaints and never objected; he suggested that she gently ask them to phone the physician on call. Dr. G. thought that she had to respond to all requests without hesitation or protest. Her self-esteem was so shaky that she was convinced she had no right to demand anything for herself or even set limits to what she should have to give. She thought the only alternative to passive acceptance was "furious anger," tantamount to homicidal rage. Week after week, Dr. G's husband would ask her, "What's more important? Your work or your family?"

After completing her residency, Dr. G. took a job with a health maintenance organization clinic, largely to please her husband and ease the marital tension by working more regular hours. She was finished each day by 5 or 6 p.m., but found herself looking for excuses to stay later. She entered psychotherapy when she became aware that she was uncomfortable spending time with her husband and children at home and longed for the hectic activity of her life as a resident. She told her therapist, "If I'm not a selfless superwoman, I feel no one will

value me." The therapist asked whether she wanted her husband
to value her. She acknowledged that the opinion of her colleagues
was more important. As the therapy progressed, Dr. G. began to
see that she was a workaholic; work sustained her hope that she
would someday receive the approval she felt she had never
received as a child. She also gained insight into her choice of
medicine as a career. The grueling pace of her residency had not
been imposed by her training director; it was a preference in
keeping with her psychological needs.

Of course, it takes two to engage in marital conflict. Physicians' spouses are harder to generalize about than physicians.
Some spouses confront compulsiveness with shrill demands for
more time, more help around the house, and more emotional availability—demands that may cause the physician to retreat into
work or search for a more sympathetic spouse elsewhere. The
second most common complaint of physicians in our survey was
that their spouses did not empathize with the demands of their
professional role and position.

Other spouses complain in a different way. They contain the
rage they feel over being neglected, but store up the day's concerns
about job, household, and children until the physician comes home.
While the physician tries to relax, the spouse recites a litany of
complaints, all of which seem to demand immediate attention.
The physician, who has already spent the day listening to complaints, may tune out by watching television, falling asleep, or
daydreaming while the spouse talks. This familiar pattern gives
rise to two of the chief complaints of spouses in our survey, namely,
that their physician spouses did not talk or listen to them. Our
findings reaffirm Goldberg's (1975) series of cases.

Still other spouses choose to suffer in silence and cling to the
fantasy that things will be better in the future. Eventually they
become disillusioned and resentful. Some glory in the role of the
long-suffering martyr; others seethe with resentment and reject
sexual advances as a way of expressing anger. Thus physicians in
our survey said that their wives' lack of interest in sex was their
main complaint. The male physician wants to make love at the
moment when his wife wants to talk.

The vocation of medicine is suited to a certain defensive style
of relating to others. At the office, physicians feel in control. They
conduct relationships with colleagues and patients on their own
terms, keeping a comfortable emotional distance. Care is given to
others but not to oneself. The same defensive style is carried into

the home. The physician wants nurturance without emotional intimacy. This puts extraordinary demands on the spouse. It is as though the physician is saying, "Take care of my dependency needs, but don't make me aware of them." The doctor wants to be fed, watered, respected, and appreciated without giving emotionally. The spouse may have to complain about physical ailments to get some attention. Then the doctor can respond by giving care from a safe emotional distance. One day the doctor realizes that he or she has married a patient, as Vaillant et al. (1972) noted. In other words, a doctor–patient or parent–child relationship was there implicitly from the beginning of the marriage. That was why the physician felt comfortable enough to make a commitment.

Another frequent complaint of spouses in Goldberg's (1975) study was that their physician husbands were too authoritarian and controlling, and treated them more like children or patients than equals. Woody Allen's joke comes to mind: "It was partially my fault we got divorced. I had a tendency to place my wife under a pedestal." The physician who hears this complaint may feel frustrated because the spouse will not be controlled by the carefully constructed defensive style that works so well in the office. Someone who ought to be grateful and appreciative is instead complaining and demanding. Like an ungrateful, litigious patient, the spouse has shattered the physician's illusions of perfection.

Conclusion

Obviously there are nonneurotic reasons for pursuing a medical career: an opportunity to be of service to others, prestige, money. We have been concerned with less conscious motivations. Although these dynamics may not be characteristic of all physicians, the vast majority should recognize something of themselves in these pages.

Surgeons as a group may be less prone to obsessive doubt and guilt feelings than other specialists such as internists, pediatricians, psychiatrists, and family practitioners. They are much more action-oriented and more likely to externalize blame. (These are only generalizations, which may or may not apply to any individual surgeon. In fact, several surgeons have told us that they think surgeons are more compulsive than internists.) Gender differences are also important. Although the cases of Dr. B., Dr. G., and the married pediatricians demonstrate that female physicians can be every bit as compulsive as males, there are also unique aspects of female psychology to be considered. They are discussed in detail in Chapters 6 and 7.

In the normal medical marriage, conflict is inevitable. Some husbands and wives give up efforts to resolve it and retreat into solitary alienation or quiet desperation. But many medical couples find ways of compromising and adapting that allow them to forge a gratifying and meaningful bond. We will have more to say about treatment and prevention in Chapters 11 and 12. The first step, however, is for both partners to understand what makes physicians the way they are.

—4—

Traditional Marriages

Roy W. Menninger, M.D.
Glen O. Gabbard, M.D.

In considering the varieties of medical marriage, we shall begin with the familiar constellation of male physician and female homemaker-wife-mother. We refer to this as the "traditional" marriage because historically it has been prevalent. As more women enter the work force, dual-career marriages may soon become more common than traditional ones. In Owens' (1966) survey, 8 percent of physicians' wives were employed outside the home; more than 20 years later, our survey indicated that 60 percent were. Nevertheless, the traditional paradigm still describes a vast number of medical marriages, particularly if we include couples in which the wife works part-time or as a volunteer.

The feature that most clearly defines this traditional marriage is a division of labor. The physician is the primary breadwinner. His domain is the office and the hospital; the wife's turf is the home and children. We will first describe how these marriages develop and then identify some of the major conflicts that arise.

The Evolution of the Traditional Marriage

From the outset, husband and wife view the marriage differently. The man regards it as a way to fulfill physical, sexual, and nutritional rather than emotional needs. Marriage provides someone to manage the kitchen, the household, and the nonmedical aspects of his life. At best, it should help him to prosper; at the least, it should "take care of itself" with little emotional support from him—even when there are children. The wife is left to tie up loose ends, and especially, to make up for what is missing because of her husband's preoccupation with training and later with medical practice.

For the wife, marriage may promise much more: a companion for life's journey, prestige and social status, enviable material comfort, and financial security. Marrying a doctor may be the fulfillment of a dream. As one satisfied wife put it, "You can be just as happily married to a rich man as you can to a poor man, so why not marry a rich man?" Many traditional wives bask in the reflected glory of their husbands.

In the earliest years, the exuberance of youth and the freshness of the dream usually sustain both partners. The doctor's "25-hour day" commitment to medicine has already begun to dominate his marriage as well as his life, displacing other activities and responsibilities, and creating an emotional environment in which pleasure, fun, and satisfaction must always be deferred. In response, both physician and spouse, but especially the spouse, speak a refrain that is part promise, part consolation, part prayer, and part hope: "Things will be better after medical school," ". . . after residency," ". . . after all his training is completed," ". . . when we are finally settled in practice"—when "life" can really begin. The repeatedly delayed gratification reflects a deeply rooted psychology of postponement in both physician and spouse, and it reinforces the physician's self-sacrificing, masochistic tendencies. Even when delay is no longer necessary, spontaneous gratification will still be difficult.

Meanwhile the wife, encouraged by social convention to accept being a helpmeet as a noble role, becomes a support system. This traditional function is exemplified in a story of the eighteenth-century surgeon, Dr. John Abernethy. As reported by Scarlett (1965):

> While attending a most respectable widow, [Dr. Abernethy]. . . became much interested in her only daughter. When the great doctor made his final visit, he took the young lady aside, and in a courtly professional tone said to her: "I have witnessed your devotion and kindness to your mother. I am in need of a wife, and I think you are the very person that would suit me. My time is incessantly occupied, and I have therefore no leisure for courting. Reflect upon this matter until Monday." She did, and subsequently became Mrs. Abernethy. But alas! there is no sequel to the story. (p. 351)

Several published commentaries describing what the physician's wife must anticipate exemplify the attitude that she has no other functions but supporting her physician husband, managing the household, and rearing the children. Terhune (1947) outlined in detail eight desirable characteristics of the physician's wife, summarized as follows: The ideal physician's wife is an attractive, intelligent, friendly, graceful, well-rounded, anonymous, strong, dedicated, and domesticated woman with stamina and forbearance. Reflecting the chauvinism of the times, his words give no hint that these expectations might be excessive, or that successful marriage requires reciprocity.

Doctors have had little to say about their "silent partners." Scarlett (1965) noted: "No doctor seems to have written a sonnet to his wife; no medical biography . . . contains . . . those touching words, . . . 'without whom I could not have done my life's work,' etc." (p. 352). Terhune (1947) is one exception. After his astonishingly bald recital of the self-sacrificing, saintly qualities required in a physician's wife, he concludes:

> I wish to express to you, in the name of the entire medical profession, the affection, admiration and gratitude which all of us feel for you, the handmaidens of medicine. We humbly acknowledge a debt which we can never repay, even were we the supermen we are not. We grant our many failings, as husbands, and realizing that we will seldom correct these failings, throw ourselves on your mercy and love. (p. 580)

Unfortunately, the passing years only reinforce the early pattern. The wife's dedicated support over many years does not make the physician more devoted to her needs or the children's. Career demands come first, last, and always. Nothing has higher priority: not their wedding anniversary, not the wife's depression, not his son's little league championship game, or even his daughter's graduation from high school. The spouse gradually realizes that nothing will change; she will remain primarily responsible for all the nonmedical aspects of the medical family, and for her personal needs as well.

Barrand (1979) observed, "[M]edicine . . . is an impeccably discreet mistress whose courtship brings approbation, acclamation, and the slow insidious destruction of relationships at home" (p. 667). For the doctor's wife, the hegemony of medicine is painful and disillusioning. As reported by Smith (1980), 70 percent of physicians' wives envision themselves as helpmeets, but more than 50 percent are disappointed in their marriages. They feel that they have made compromises (64 percent) and that they have suffered from the physician's "god" status (48.2 percent). Nevertheless, 67.7 percent felt they had achieved their goal.

Medical practice becomes ascendant despite avowals that it cannot or will not or must not. This results from a pervasive conflict between the moral imperatives of good medical practice and the moral imperatives of marriage and family. Despite good intentions, many physicians cannot make room for both.

Time further demonstrates the hidden cost of that convenient division of labor, as it inexorably leads to diverging courses of growth and patterns of living. The physician and his wife become more and more distant, less and less intimate. Eventually the marriage may be emptied of vitality and warmth, sustained only by economic obligations.

The marriage has gone wrong because, as our survey shows, physician and spouse have differing perceptions of the problems in the marriage, differing needs for intimacy, differing styles of communication, and vastly different unexpressed expectations.

Gender Differences

Gilligan (1982) has eloquently described how gender differences affect the development of identity. To establish a masculine identity, boys must develop autonomy by separating themselves from their mothers. Separation and autonomy are not so important for girls; their female identities can develop in close association with their mothers. Thus boys seek independence and self-sufficiency; girls seek relatedness and emotional closeness. Girls develop a capacity for empathy because establishment of clear boundaries between themselves and their mothers is not as psychologically urgent as it is for males. As Gilligan put it:

> Since masculinity is defined through separation while femininity is defined through attachment, male gender identity is threatened by intimacy while female gender identity is threatened by separation. Thus males tend to have difficulty with relationships, while females tend to have problems with individuation. (p. 8)

Thus the male physician expects and desires much less intimacy in marriage than does his wife, as our Chapter 2 study confirms.

> One traditional physician couple, Clark and Betty, illustrate this common source of tension. Clark was a 39-year-old endocrinologist, and Betty a 37-year-old homemaker. At their

first session of marital therapy, the therapist asked them to describe their problems. Betty complained that Clark was never home in time for supper with her and the children; Clark complained that Betty did not appreciate the demands of a busy medical practice. He said that he had built his reputation by listening to patients and spending time with them, and simply could not rush through rounds to get home by 6 p.m. Betty insisted that the demands of his practice were not really the issue. "Even when Clark is home," she complained, "he doesn't want to spend time with me." Clark exploded, feeling unjustly accused. "All she wants to do is watch television," explained Clark. "I hate television. I like to read." Betty's idea of spending time together was to sit together on the couch, cuddle, and chat about their day's activities as they watched television. Clark's idea of spending time together was his reading in one room while Betty read in another. Betty said she could not remember a single time in the last year when the two of them had done something together for fun. Clark objected, mentioning several evenings when they had gone sailing with friends. Betty said that she did not consider that doing something together. Clark insisted that they were doing something together even if friends were along too. As the result of these tensions, Clark persistently distanced himself by staying away from home and refusing to tell Betty where he was. Betty in turn pursued him with phone calls, interrupting him repeatedly all over town.

Marital therapy brought them to see how radically different were their expectations and needs for intimacy. Betty came to see the problem as her need for much more emotional intimacy with Clark than he could give; Clark came to define the problem as his need for more freedom and "space" than Betty could tolerate.

This couple also alluded to their deepest fears as they revealed their needs for intimacy or distance. Gilligan (1982) used projective psychological testing (the Thematic Apperception Test) to study male–female differences in hidden fears and fantasies. She found that men were likely to attribute risk to personal affiliation, while achievement and competition seemed risky to women:

> The danger men describe in their stories of intimacy is a danger of entrapment or betrayal, being caught in a smothering relationship or humiliated by rejection and deceit. In contrast, the danger women portray in their tales of achievement is a danger of isolation, a fear that in standing out or being set apart by success, they will be left alone. (p. 42)

These findings further illuminate the causes of the impasse in Clark and Betty's marriage. Clark saw in Betty's demand for emotional closeness a threat of humiliation, entrapment, and smothering. Betty saw in his need for distance a threat that she would be abandoned and left totally alone.

Since the issue is usually presented in the guise of problems about time, neither husband nor wife is readily able to see the conflict for what it really is. Even the children may be used by the doctor as convenient barriers to intimacy. One doctor's wife described the problem as follows:

> My husband's relationship with the kids is a problem for me. He adores them but in a kind of glommed-on [sic] undifferentiated way. There is no space for him and me to be two adults with an adult sexual relationship. We cannot have a conversation that the kids don't interrupt. When they do interrupt, *they* always have his full attention, not me. It is infuriating. He and the kids are a unit, and I often feel like an outsider. I think my husband's kind of permissive, undifferentiated relationship with our children is going to be a real factor in our eventual divorce—as well as his deeply sensitive, but just kind of closed-off, way of relating to me and the world.

The doctor is likely to feel guilty about how little time he spends with his children. He may try to make up for this (and salve his conscience) by interacting with his wife and children in a pressured, somewhat artificial and occasionally autocratic way. Instead of pleasing everyone, he usually pleases no one: he remains preoccupied, only partially attentive or impatient, looking forward to the moment when he can turn to something else. The interaction—and the intimacy that should be part of it—is unsatisfying at best and distasteful at worst. He is usually quite unconscious of using his children as a means of avoiding intimacy with his wife; he may be amazed and even annoyed at the suggestion. Consciously, he is only playing the role of a devoted father.

Impairments of Communication

Problems with emotional intimacy often become problems in communication. Women are much more comfortable sharing their feelings; they are more relationship- and "togetherness"-oriented, and find satisfaction in the interactions themselves. Men are often reluctant to talk with their wives if it carries the risk of emotional involvement. As our Chapter 2 findings reflect, the main complaint of doctors' wives is that their husbands do not talk to them. One psychiatrist's wife described her situation as follows:

The biggest drawback to intimacy in our marriage is that my husband does not share his thoughts and feelings much. He plays psychiatrist at home instead of [being] one of the family. He is loving and supportive of *my* sharing, but he is always distant. He tunes out at will when sharing is important.

As we have pointed out in Chapter 3, the male physician is likely to be emotionally constricted to begin with, and that constriction is reinforced by medical training.

Bill is a 47-year-old internist, and Alice a 44-year-old home-maker. He has tried to explain to her that he simply cannot talk to her in the way she wants him to. He poignantly states: "I just don't know how. I don't think I can ever change that." When he is under stress at work or feeling depressed, he becomes even more silent and reserved. He feels strongly that anger at work can never be justified, and does everything in his power to avoid it. He showed no anger even when a hospital nurse verbally abused one of his relatives before his eyes. When he comes home, Alice suffers from the frustration that he has built up during the day. She feels ignored as he sulks and silently fumes around the house. At bedtime Bill expects her to make love, even though he hasn't said two words to her all evening.

This marital dance reflects a fundamental difference in gender-related styles of communication. As one female colleague summarized it: "Men talk so that they can make love; women make love so they can talk" (S. J. Larson, personal communication, 1986). Each marital partner "knows" what the other wants, and that knowledge provides a convenient weapon in marital dueling. When she is angry, she withholds sex. When he is angry, he withholds conversation. If the wife withholds sex, she is likely to feel guilty later because she is so acutely aware of how little pleasure her husband gets. One wife described her marriage as follows:

The tension is there for me without doubt, but there is little if any verbal conflict. Anger and conflict I withdraw from. In the past he's expressed such discouragement that I rarely say anything. I also don't want to hurt him. There seems to be very little in life that gives him pleasure. I feel on the whole I've been little help to him.

These words betray the sense of failure that is often felt by the traditional wife. She has taken on the role of support system with great enthusiasm, but finds she can do little to give her husband pleasure. He always seems overburdened, tense, and consumed by work. Many wives assume that they are doing something wrong.

The marital partners may go on living for many years without overt conflict, each speaking a different language, neither hearing the other's pleas. Often it takes a crisis such as a malpractice suit to bring conflicts into the open. One 52-year-old family practitioner recalled:

> We did very well the first 6 years of our marriage, before we had our first child and before I was involved as a solo practitioner in a small town. We then grew apart as I was totally engrossed in my practice and she was busy with our three young children. The great stress that demonstrated our growing hostility and separation from each other was a lawsuit that dragged on over 3 years. It was devastating to me psychologically; and when I turned to her, I felt I did not get any support. I was only then aware of how angry she actually was with me. We went to marital counseling, but the tension in our relationship remained high with considerable anger and hostility. We fell into a common pattern. I spent money on investments, which she resented. She was not particularly warm or affectionate or sexually receptive, which I resented. If we had not gone to counseling, I am sure we would have been irrevocably alienated.

These comments illustrate the remarkable capacity of many physicians to remain oblivious to their spouses' feelings. Until he turned to his wife in a crisis, he was completely unaware of her seething anger. The malpractice suit did not *cause* the tension in the marriage; it had been building for years, while the physician functioned on "automatic pilot," paying no attention to his wife's verbal and nonverbal messages. The malpractice suit changed the rules of the game. For the first time in years, he turned to his wife for emotional support, and was surprised to find that she would not give him what he had denied her. When communication has been nonexistent or limited, a traumatic event like a lawsuit creates demands that are impossible to satisfy. Each member of the couple feels as though transported to a foreign country with no knowledge of the native language.

In marriages that are essentially solid and mutually rewarding, the partners can usually manage a good deal of conflict. But a malpractice suit can threaten even the most durable of marriages.

Phil, a highly respected 56-year-old surgeon, and Nan, also 56, a homemaker, had been happily married for 25 years when Phil was sued for malpractice. He was taken completely by surprise, and was devastated when the news was published in the local newspaper. His colleagues said nothing to him about the suit, and he was haunted by fantasies about what they were thinking. He lost all interest in sex and had severe insomnia for months. Nan begged him to talk with her about his fears; instead he brought home copies of depositions for her to read. Nan dutifully read them, but felt that she was not doing enough to support him.

After the suit was successfully resolved, Phil commented that his self-esteem had never been very high, but through diligent, conscientious work, he had gradually developed a conviction that he was a competent physician. To maintain this sense of himself, he needed regular indications that his work was good and that others appreciated and respected it. The suit itself was a devastating attack on his self-image. The silence of his colleagues seemed to confirm that negative view, leaving him at the mercy of his latent fears and doubts. He felt that talking about these painful feelings, even with his wife, would only further undermine his shaky self-confidence. Sharing the depositions was his way of involving her without having to talk about it openly. Later when asked whether he had shared his worst fears with Nan, Phil evaded the question with the comment, "I think she knew my worst fears."

Phil's response to this question is telling from another perspective. Nelson (1978) suggested that the language of the physician is the language of logic, and that the language of his wife is the language of emotion. But the logic may be only superficial; in his response Phil conveyed a highly illogical form of magical thinking. He expected his wife to know what he was thinking (and feeling) without his having to tell her. He also thought that if he did not talk about the fears, they would somehow be less justified, less real, and therefore less threatening.

Dependence on mind reading and the magical avoidance of danger is decidedly unrealistic. What is worse, this strategy diminishes the relationship and deprives both parties of the substantial emotional support that each wants, and wants to provide to the other. In a similar way physicians often expect their emotional needs to be taken care of without having to ask their spouses. This is a source of frustration for the spouse. A wife can see that she is not fulfilling her husband's needs, but he does little to help her learn how; the dutiful wife is reduced to guessing.

The diagnosis of the problem as lack of communication is perhaps misleading. In fact, everyone communicates; one can't *not* communicate. Actions may replace words, but communicating goes on. Not showing up for dinner, for example, without calling is still a communication. What couples usually mean by this phrase is that they don't like what a marital partner is communicating. Independent written accounts by a doctor and his wife from our questionnaire survey in Chapter 2 represent a familiar situation of this sort. The physician describes the problems as follows:

> She would state that our problems relate to deficiencies of communication. She would say that we never talk to each other about significant relations. I would state that our problem is the inability to agree on, understand, work on, talk about, share, spend time on, enjoy, strive for, common goals and objectives. However, our marriage will last until death do us part, because of the obligation we assumed, beginning with the marriage vows, our families, our five children, and the expectations of society. Our marriage will probably improve with time, as I achieve the goals and objectives that I have felt important, and have time to do the things my wife would like to do. Time is really the issue. I can communicate better when there is time to do it. There would be fewer problems if I could follow a time schedule that I have written, but haven't been able to follow.

The wife's version:

> Knowing my husband doesn't like me very well is not exactly conducive to feeling comfortable. I can't share my feelings with him because he doesn't make me feel any better. He is just determined to make this marriage work somehow, but love has *nothing* to do with it. Everything and everybody (especially children) should be spic-and-span most of the time. I keep trying to think of something I can do well (in his eyes), but there isn't much. Thank goodness I get good reinforcement from some friends and acquaintances to maintain my self-esteem. There are times I see a glimmer of caring beginning to develop, so I keep hoping that it will develop into a meaningful relationship. It definitely has improved in the last year, and we have had more "ups" than "downs." It is just that I long so for that good feeling of being loved again, and occasionally it catches up with me and I get teary eyed.

Each partner is hoping against hope that things will ultimately get better. Meanwhile they live lives of quiet desperation.

Male physicians are often remarkably inarticulate and sphinx-like on any topic relating to the marital relationship—how he feels about it, or what his wife might be feeling or thinking about it. Although he may believe it is a loving relationship, he is often quite unable to say how he knows that, or how either of them conveys love to the other. Such a physician tends to talk about the relationship in intellectualized terms, as if he were discussing a clinical problem with a colleague. His wife, on the other hand, may be the one who identifies the problems and insists on change. As the spokesperson for the feelings of the couple, she may show the pain in the relationship with grimaces, dismay, obvious discouragement, and even tears.

This intellectual/affective division of communication often reflects long-standing personality differences, and can be self-perpetuating. With endless repetition, each comes to know the "scripts" of the other, and each becomes less able or willing to understand or empathize with the other. When such patterns of split communication become entrenched, the possibility of change, even in a desired direction, raises new anxiety and strong resistance.

The discovery that the communication difficulty is bilateral can be a surprise, since each is usually convinced that the problem lies in the other. The experiences of Joan and John illustrate the point:

> The truth can be painful. For years I blamed John for not wanting to share feelings and for getting caught up in his routine at the expense of our relationship. After a week in Colorado [at the Physicians and Their Families Workshop] I saw real change in him. He was more willing to share feelings, but I didn't always want to hear them. He was trying to reset priorities, and I was the one more comfortable with old routines. All week [at the workshop] the doctor is told that his rational, organized training and thought processes are okay for his medical practice but not good for his personal relationships. If he takes this to heart, as John did, and attempts to change, I think the spouse's possible resistance should also be taken into account. I do not know if I was more willing to share feelings when we were first married, but after 16 years of marriage and believing it was John, not me, my discovery was somewhat shocking. Now at least, I am just as much, if not more responsible for maintaining the status quo.

A Vicarious Identity

In our Chapter 2 survey, the second most common complaint of wives about their husbands was, "He doesn't provide enough emotional support for me." This is the familiar lament of the traditional wife, who feels that her husband gives to everyone else all day and has nothing left to give to her. Other women at the supermarket go on and on about her husband's many virtues, while she secretly thinks, "If they only knew." She was attracted to him in the first place partly because he was so obviously a caring, loving, and giving person, someone who had dedicated his life to serving humanity. But when she sits down with him to share her concerns, his eyes glaze over as he tunes her out on the way to falling asleep.

One wife describes it this way: "Even when he's with me, he's not really there." The physician thinks about his work obsessively every waking minute. While his wife is telling him about the dishwasher malfunction, he is thinking about whether he should have done a lumbar puncture on the child he saw in the emergency room. This tendency to avoid listening by ruminating about clinical matters serves a powerful defensive function. He avoids intense emotional contact with his wife, diminishing the bond between them; repetition without change may eventually lead her to give up even trying to communicate with him.

This familiar situation creates another source of tension in traditional medical marriages. The husband feels that he is selflessly devoting himself to his patients, while the wife accuses him of being selfish and inconsiderate. A classic example is the case of an obstetrician's wife whose husband was delivering their baby until he was called away to attend another patient in a different delivery room. His wife was left to be delivered by the nurse, while he "selflessly" cared for the other patient.

After years without emotional support from her husband, the traditional wife may come to believe that her activities and concerns are no longer *legitimate*. That view is strongly reinforced by the general social judgment that household maintenance by wives is not "work" and that homemakers deserve low status because they are not producers (Crawford and Lorch 1981). Domestic matters do not seem to matter to the one who counts most: her husband. She is never allowed to forget that these tasks are trivial compared to his pressing medical decisions about life and death.

So the wife's identity becomes dependent on the identity of her husband; Zemon-Gass and Nichols (1975) called this the "take me along" marital syndrome. Her identity is contingent, a reflection of her husband's accomplishments and prestige; she is "Mrs. *John* Smith," not Jane Smith.

The traditional attitudes of others reinforce this denial of individuality. This was graphically illustrated by the experience of the wife of a prominent physician. She had been asked to address the wives of a professional group, and her husband came along as her escort. Her name badge, however, read "Mrs. *James* Jones," while her husband's erroneously read "Dr. James Jones, SPEAKER."

Wives with a contingent identity learn to be passive, to sustain a noncomplaining self-sacrificial attitude, and to forsake personal ambition; they become persons without aims beyond those defined by the role as wife and mother. One wife describes it this way:

> The amount of time he spends away from home in nonpatient-care activities seems to be preventing me from returning to work. His concern seems to be that I won't be available for vacations. He prefers that I continue to do volunteer work. I realize that I could never match his earning capacity, but I would feel like a contributor to our home by bringing in a paycheck for doing what I enjoy instead of cutting grass and washing dishes.

This sense of isolation and low self-esteem has increased greatly now that most households have two full-time earners. Many traditional wives are embarrassed about being "mere homemakers"; they admit it defensively and apprehensively.

The risks of such a limited and negative sense of self are considerable. Traditional wives are already economically dependent on their husbands. Their sense of inferiority may intensify these dependent needs and further reduce their capacity for autonomous action. This may lead to functional helplessness, and eventually, overt manifestations of illness. Miles et al.'s (1975) finding of a high incidence of marital turmoil in hospitalized physicians' wives suggests that a wife's illness may be a symptom of a troubled marriage. Vincent (1969) and Schoicket (1978), among others, have observed that symptoms requiring medications, even intravenous or intramuscular injections, fulfill certain emotional needs of the wife, her physician husband, and the relationship itself. As a patient, she receives her husband's attention in however inadequate a form. He provides that attention in a way that assuages his guilt by relieving her physical discomfort, while ignoring its psychological roots; and this interaction sustains the relationship at a neurotic level fraught with strong feelings of dependency, resentment, self-pity, guilt, and anger.

The middle years of the marriage may bring to the wife feelings of sadness and emptiness intensified by the departure of her children and the consequent loss of one of her most important and fulfilling roles. If she cannot replace it with a role that both she and her husband consider significant, deficiencies in the marital relationship itself may precipitate illness in the form of alcoholism, drug dependence, hypochondriasis, and above all, depression.

To avoid the vicissitudes of a contingent identity, the traditional medical wife must become something more than a homemaker and mother. In the next chapter, Bev Menninger discusses this problem and some ways to resolve it.

Perspective of a Medical Wife: Surviving on the Edge of the Spotlight

Bev Menninger

As the foregoing chapters have shown, the physician's wife lives in a world whose attractive appearance is often belied by the silent and subtle inner constraints produced by her husband's personality and practice.

The options of response are also limited, particularly for women whose first priority is sustaining a successful marriage. Most physicians' wives have one thing in common: their husbands are the primary wage earners, the pivotal figures in the family and the community, the one in the spotlight. Traditional wives are almost always at the edge of that spotlight.

That is, of course, exactly where most of them have chosen to be, and certainly most assume from the outset that that is where they will be. Especially in economically uncertain times, physicians' wives may feel so privileged to be married to old-fashioned good providers that they suppress any urge to voice dissatisfaction or doubt.

The advantages of being married to an ambitious, high-achieving husband usually outweigh the disadvantages. These benefits include a comfortable standard of living, relative freedom from financial worries, and often the option to stay home to rear children or to pursue personal interests. Most traditional wives would not trade these advantages for whatever satisfactions and demands a spotlighted career of their own might bring. Maybe that is why some women, when encouraged to discuss their frustrations, become quite defensive or *very quiet*. It is as if talking about or even acknowledging the inevitable difficulties is criticism of or a threat to their husbands or their marriages. Yet refusing to air grievances and failing to work toward an acceptable balance in marriage is inherently dangerous.

Because they are always the "support system," never the star, wives are often overlooked, pushed aside, or ignored altogether in the rush to sit at the feet of their husbands. They must adjust to subordinating their own needs to those of their husbands and children, as they vigorously, sometimes frantically, seek to be an adequate support system for the family. It is not easy; it is sometimes not very pleasant; nor is it avoidable in the circumstances.

I knew I would be on the edge of a spotlight before I married Roy. You couldn't grow up in the Midwest and not know of the Menninger family. My initiation occurred the day before our wedding, when he did a symposium with one of our trustees, Margaret Mead, in New York. The next day we were married in Topeka; the day after he was on the Merv Griffin show in Hollywood. He, of course, thought that justified his later comment (at a particularly difficult time) that I knew what I was getting into. Maybe so, but after my reaction, he won't soon say it again!

On another occasion I discovered I wasn't prepared for my reception as Roy's wife at a dinner party we were giving for Menninger trustees and contributors at a large Los Angeles hotel. He asked me to be on the lookout for a certain woman he knew would be coming to the party alone. When I spotted her, I walked up, introduced myself, and welcomed her to the party. She looked me up and down and then said, "Well, you're not *really* a Menninger!" When I asked what she meant, she said, "Well, you're not a daughter or a sister!" For once I had my wits about me and replied, "No, I'm one of the chosen ones." She avoided me for the rest of the evening, but later she took Roy aside and invited him to lunch with her, alone, to receive a generous donation. Much to his credit— in my eyes at least!—he delegated that lunch to the director of development.

Of course each physician's wife has different experiences, but others may feel similar dismay and irritation when they are ignored while their physician husbands are immediately corralled at social gatherings for "off-the-cuff" advice.

Risks and Hazards

Being on the edge of the spotlight means facing these awkward and sometimes irritating experiences repeatedly—and they are funny only in the retelling. There is a price to be paid for marriage to a high-powered man: some hazards, some distressing costs, and, most troubling of all, some risks to mental health.

The first risk of being on the edge is the husband's and wife's diverging activity tracks. Unless they make specific efforts to prevent it, they will be inexorably carried further and further apart by the natural course of events and the passage of time.

The physician invests more and more time and energy in his career, usually at the expense of time spent with his wife and family. His wife finds fewer and fewer opportunities to participate in the excitement and challenge of her husband's world, even vicariously. Her responsibilities at home leave little time for that, and he shares his work world with her less as it becomes more complex and absorbing. As the physician increasingly finds his needs for attention, appreciation, and intimacy met by his work, his colleagues, and his patients, his psychological need for his wife is diminished. The marriage may gradually become an "arrangement," and less and less one of love. This progressive disengagement may only become apparent during the middle years, when the husband, having dedicated his life to his occupation and his identity as a physician, awakens to a long unmet need for intimacy. On the other hand, after years of providing nurturance and intimacy in her role as mother and wife, his wife has discovered the possibilities for a more distinctive identity, and begins to pursue it. Husband and wife pass each other like ships in the night (Figure 1). Yet it's nobody's fault. *Each* is only doing what he or she is programmed to do. *Each* now looks for what they've missed.

This deterioration has been likened to the school laboratory experiment of killing a frog. Dropping it into boiling water won't work; it immediately jumps out. But if you put it in a pan of cool water and gradually heat it, the frog is cooked before it realizes the danger. Partners on diverging tracks who *do not* make efforts to reconnect during the busiest years may find that their marriage, like the frog, is slowly dying.

Figure 1. Midlife Crossover Pattern in the Traditional Marriage

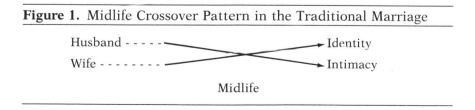

Jane, a childhood friend, told me about the slow deterioration and tragic outcome of her parents' marriage. Although her father was not a physician, the pattern is similar.

My parents were married very young. When my father began his business, my mother was his bookkeeper and better educated than he. She could discuss his new ventures with him quite competently. He looked to her for help, and was a major part of his support during his early years. He was remarkably successful. But as his company expanded, he traveled more and more.

Because Mother was increasingly needed as a hostess to entertain my father's business associates and his important customers, she quit her bookkeeping job. At the same time, there was less and less sharing of ideas about his plans for expansion. This was partly because he was gone so much, and partly because he was beginning to feel more important and more powerful, and even superior to her.

But what was worse was the fact that he now had an efficient, attractive, attentive, and ambitious female executive assistant who, of course, knew his business very well, was eager to discuss it with him, always there, and very much afraid to argue with him since her job was on the line. Mother, on the other hand, did not agree with everything he did, and was not reluctant to say so. When she did, he turned back to his assistant who was there to "lick his wounds."

With his continuing success, power and money began to take precedence over everything (and everyone) else; getting ahead was the only important thing. Then disaster hit. He lost control of his company, and suddenly the power and the spotlight were gone. Now he was angry. He had been distant from his family for years, but with no target for his anger, he turned on us and blamed us for everything: his failure was our fault, we weren't supportive enough, we demanded too much, we didn't do the right things, and on and on. In the face of such vituperation, Mother found it impossible to continue. Her plans to file for divorce after 37 years of marriage were interrupted only when he suddenly had a fatal heart attack.

As this example suggests, without continuing efforts to stay connected, women and their successful husbands will find it virtually impossible to avoid the ultimate destruction of their marriages. Prevention is the only answer.

Responding to her high-achieving husband with a competitive need to do as well is *the second risk* faced by the wife of a busy, pressured, active husband. Caught up in the high-demand atmosphere of a professional marriage, such a wife tries to be model wife, perfect mother, and a successful career woman as well. It means being a gourmet cook, able to entertain beautifully and uncomplainingly on short notice, occasionally acting as both host and hostess because her husband is still with a patient or finishing paperwork. It means having sufficient understanding of—and patience with—the nature of his business so that he can discuss its problems with her and not *always* with someone else. And, of course, it means being well-groomed and charming at all times.

It means being not just a good mother, but also president of the PTA, active in the medical auxiliary, chairperson of the state committee on child abuse, as well as head of the parents' council on art in the schools and the local ballet group. Even for ambitious, high-energy women, this guarantees pressure: trying to live up to everyone's idea of competence, while also trying to decide what kind of person you want to be when you aren't busy being somebody's wife, or somebody's daughter, or somebody's mother.

Such a wife is at risk for burning out, feeling overwhelmed and inadequate, and failing to live up even to her own expectations, much less those of her family. Moreover, there is no good way to cry "stop," short of breaking down, flying apart, or falling flat. Have you ever become sick and thought, "At least *now* I can get a rest!"? Taking time for oneself incurs guilt in most of us; illness is often the only acceptable excuse for slowing down or stopping.

The third risk results from the effects of the spotlight on the physician husband. Being regarded as all-powerful and shouldering life-and-death responsibilities can make him lose humility, sometimes to the point of altering personality. Surrounded by compliant hospital and office personnel (often young, attractive, and female), respected by friends and social acquaintances, and admired by strangers, the spotlighted physician husband may begin to believe he is as good, as effective, as competent, as noble, as intelligent as his public thinks he is. With dismay and rising indignation, the wife may watch as the fluttering females flock to pay homage to the star—and he eats it up! Some physicians expect the same worshipful treatment at home from their wives and children, and they may feel deprived and irritated, even hurt, when it is not forthcoming. It may be very difficult for physicians' wives to keep a picture of reality before their husbands and to work to keep them humble.

Responses to Living at the Edge of the Spotlight

Three of the most common responses to these stresses and hazards are: (*1*) the support system, (*2*) an independent career, and (*3*) the creative compromise.

The *support system* response is the traditional pattern. It often requires total compliance with the family's demands. In this role, a woman must often suppress both her negative reactions of irritation and her positive aspirations for creativity, telling herself that her turn will come later—after the children start school, after the children leave home, maybe after her husband retires. This fond hope assumes one's readiness for that future when it arrives and takes no account of the froglike death that may supervene.

> Susan's husband, a surgeon, was absolutely single-minded; his goal in life was simply to build his practice as fast and as big as he could. She agreed that he would make the money and she would take care of everything else—rearing the children, making a home, community involvement, and church responsibilities. They would have few social engagements or vacations until they had made it. By age 45, most of the sacrifices had been made; they had built a new home and were planning their first long trip—alone and without the children. Susan told me this when I went to visit her after her husband's funeral. After they had made reservations for the cruise, he had had a heart attack. She had discovered that during all those years she was waiting and planning, her husband had been having an affair. He evidently needed a little excitement while he waited. It does not do to live your life in the future.

Of course, the rewards of mothering help to make the support system role acceptable, at least during the earliest years. For many women, that role fits their needs and expectations quite adequately. The tacit agreement is: "I will provide a clean house, rear well-mannered and well-bred children, prepare hot dinners, and be an attractive social hostess and bed companion in return for being taken care of and protected from the outside world."

The costs of this arrangement increase with the passage of time but remain hidden until they come due. The supportive wife-mother is so busy that she becomes aware of the price only very much later.

Suddenly (or so it seems) the children are gone, and so is her husband. Probably not literally (because studies show that medical marriages have a low divorce rate despite a high degree of unhappiness), but in terms of common interests and a common life. She now asks, "Who am I?"—and often has no answer. She has paid her dues and yet has very little personal achievement or sense of identity to show for it; a successful husband and attractive children are not enough. Latent self-pity may become manifest, as well as hypochondriasis, alcoholism and drug abuse, and, above all, depression. Maggie Scarf (1980) noted:

> In every study carried out everywhere and anywhere, more women than men were in treatment for depression. It was so in every institution—inpatient and outpatient—across the country. It was true in state and county facilities, and in community mental health centers. It was simply true across the board. Even when the figures were adjusted for age, or phase of life, or social class and economic circumstances—in other words, any which way—the outcome was still the same: anywhere from two to six times as many females as males in treatment for depression. (pp. 2–3)

In dramatic contrast to this compliant style is the response of women with *independent career* aims. In recent years many married women have entered the work force, sometimes for economic reasons but sometimes also as an expression of personal interest and need. This may solve the problem of maintaining a career and a marriage at the same time—but only if such women are doing something they enjoy, rather than just getting out of the house, and only if their marital relationship is mature. A mature relationship involves genuine sharing of two lives, not just two parallel careers of two people living together. Too often, the demands of a career make even heavier demands on the marriage, and ultimately an either–or choice is forced. Many women must then either choose the career path or compromise their career advancement to keep the marriage intact.

Another option is the *creative compromise*, which provides some of the benefits of both a fulfilling marriage and growth-producing challenges that lead to a separate identity. The word *creative* suggests that this often means altering one's habits to include at least one special, perhaps new, program for oneself. Unfortunately, adding something new may not work; most lives are already very busy, and adding one thing usually means dropping or cutting back on something else.

The word *compromise* also implies compromise on the part of the physician husband. There will be times when his wife's achievements give her a moment in the spotlight and he is on the edge. When, for example, a painting of mine wins a prize or gets a good price, or when I have an exhibit and my husband attends as my "spouse," it is not a very comfortable position for him, as I've discovered!

Obstacles to Achieving a Creative Compromise

Of all the circumstances that may affect plans to achieve an "ideal" compromise, none is more critical than the attitudes and expectations of the husband. These can range from active support and participation through various kinds of ambivalence and degrees of indifference to outright hostility and active resistance to change.

Not surprisingly, the extremes of this spectrum are the easiest to manage. Even clear opposition helps to define the challenge, clarify the resistance, and permit the marital couple to "have it out" and reach a resolution. It is the ambivalence that proves hardest to manage. Too often one does not know where the other person stands and is afraid to confront the question with sufficient clarity to permit a decision.

Some wives, for example, concede defeat without protest and keep their anger bottled up until the pressure forces an explosion of some sort—a fight, an illness, or a misbehaving child. Often the husband has no clear idea how important it is for his wife to redefine herself and her interests. In the name of "protecting" him, she reinforces his continuing ignorance of her needs: but he's so busy; his job is so important; this wouldn't really add to our income but, oh, how I'd love it. It is as if asking for her husband's support and interest is demanding an unjustifiable indulgence. The resentment and guilt continue to build, and the relationship suffers from a psychological burden neither party really understands.

> Jane was a most competent artist, the wife of a respected internist. When the children were about to leave home, she decided to open a studio, teach, and sell her work and the work of her artist friends. Her husband went along, even to the extent of helping with the carpentry and plumbing in the new studio, while joking about the tax write-off it would afford. At about the same time, he assumed an administrative position with a hospital corporation and began to travel in earnest, as much as half-time. He wanted her to travel with him, but she was now busy and felt less and less inclined to go. That distressed him.

Worse, when her project began to make money, he became upset and even annoyed. A prospective failure he could tolerate (it was a tax loss, after all); her success he could not.

Jane was ominously quiet for a while. Then one day she closed the studio and began to travel with her husband. She had given up painting. It was a tremendous sacrifice for a person who needs to paint as most of us need to eat and sleep. Indeed, painting was at the core of her identity.

It became clear that all was not well. She began to hint at separation. It seemed that she had gone from doing exactly what *she* wanted to do to exactly what *he* wanted. As a result, somebody was always completely unhappy. She had clearly never considered a compromise; in fact, she wouldn't even talk about it. She had been oblivious to his increasing distress, and was caught by surprise when he finally voiced it. Since her marriage was important to her and she cared about him, she made an abrupt about-face and sought to be a full-time wife, whatever the cost to her. Soon she required a brief stay in the psychiatric ward of a general hospital. Only then, under the pressure of the crisis and at the urging of her therapist, did both of them begin to talk about their perceptions and feelings. Only then did a real compromise become possible.

Even the most liberal-minded man may have surprising feelings about his wife's success, feelings that may intensify as her success begins to demand changes in marital routines.

Karen and Bill were such a couple. He was the busy and successful president of a large company that his father had started. His home and children were in Karen's hands; she was quite capable of running the house and parts of the community as well. She soon became a leader in whatever group she became a part of, even serving as president of two at the same time. Although it was stressful for the children and for her husband, they were never neglected. After many years as a successful volunteer leader, she was ready for new challenges when her children left home.

Like so many wives, she found herself relatively unqualified for employment. Her talents as a community leader had little market appeal. She decided to go to law school. Her husband agreed, even though it meant TV dinners, less social life, and even vacation time spent apart.

Thinking of her as someone who had identified her own needs, made a decision, retained her husband's support, and successfully managed the transition from mother-homemaker to career woman without destroying her marriage, I called her to discuss these issues. I found her much less confident than she had

been at the outset. After graduating from law school and passing
the bar, she had realized that a part-time law practice isn't
possible; it had to be all or nothing. When this became clear to
her husband, he rebelled. Now that the children were gone, he
wanted to enjoy time with his wife—just as she was ready to
begin a new and very involving life. Unfortunately, matters had
gone too far; neither could continue to meet the needs of the
other, and divorce was the only solution.

It is as if some husbands see their sense of male strength and
competence as resting on the presence of an inadequate, dependent
female. A wife's self-advancement efforts are tolerable only as long
as they remain modest and hobby-like, offering no threat to the
status quo.

An example of this situation involved my friend Virginia. She
was a talented women with a masters degree who wrote and
illustrated a history book that was adopted by schools as an
elementary text. Emboldened by her success, she thought of
returning to graduate school for a doctorate. She enthusiastically
discussed these plans with her physician husband and was
entirely unprepared for his negative reaction. "No!" he said,
"there will be only one doctor in this household!" Abruptly she
abandoned her plans. "Of course," Virginia explained, "keeping
my marriage is more important than getting another degree."

One of the things that interferes with efforts to develop a
viable compromise is the wife's hesitancy to speak her thoughts
openly and to confront these issues. A streak of timidity—even
fear—runs deep in many women. For too long they have been
taught to accept a subordinate, compliant role. Asking hard questions about new opportunities or changes in the relationship is
believed to be a surefire recipe for the destruction of a marriage.
To call attention to inequities, to protest a monotonous role, to
seek a new and better personal marital adjustment is risky. But
even at its worst, the stress of confrontation and discussion is *not*
more destructive than the deterioration of spirit that comes from
a failure to satisfy personal needs for identity and worth. This kind
of confrontation with oneself and one's partner takes courage that
comes from conviction. It requires some clarity about where one
is trying to go, and some awareness of what tools and techniques
to use.

Critical Next Steps

The techniques for pursuing a creative compromise involve settling one's own issues and opening the dialogue.

The first task is perhaps the toughest. As indirect evidence of this, it is significant that many women, when asked about their problems, will list a dozen, all of which are external: in the environment, in other people, in the institutions they live and work with, in their neighbors, in their children, or even in their husbands. They practically never cite problems in themselves. But this is the only place we can start since we are the only person we have control over. It is our responsibility and no one else's.

The task is to identify the options. That means understanding just what it is we really want out of life and what we want to be remembered for. But often we have been brainwashed by instructions about what we ought to want, or have never looked carefully at what we do well and we most enjoy. As physician's wives, most of us want both a good marriage and family, *and* a sense of psychological independence and achievement. Understanding that no one can ever fully have both is an important first step, part of the creative compromise.

The physician's wife must start with a thoughtful assessment of what she does well or would like to do well. She might look first at past interests that have been set aside, something started in youth but not pursued. She may also find opportunity in a new experience that can be exploited and developed into a significant activity.

It has been that way for both me and my husband Roy. In middle age, Roy decided he would like to play in the civic symphony. He had taken cello lessons briefly as a youngster, and at the age of 40, he resumed them. Once a week he drove to another town for his lessons and made time for practice in the evenings. He didn't find the time he needed; he *made* it. After several years of work, he successfully joined the symphony. He will never be First Chair, but he has been able to enjoy a cherished dream.

About 10 years ago, my mother-in-law invited me to go to a watercolor workshop. My reply was, "I appreciate the invitation, but I haven't held a paintbrush in my hands since Prang paints in grade school!" She insisted, saying I could always take a good book, sit under a tree, and read. So I went. After the first lesson I was so excited I couldn't sleep. I found, to my continuing amazement, that somewhere within me is a talent for painting I never knew existed. It has led me into a new world of friends, new experiences, new excitements that are my very own—and a new and stronger sense of ME.

I took advantage of an opportunity, and now my paintings are hanging in exhibits, winning awards, and selling—and it feels good! What made the difference was not the experience of the workshop, however exciting. It was persisting and investing the effort it took to make that activity my own. The results: occasional failure, frequent frustration, but very important successes. It has also meant making tough choices between painting and traveling with Roy. Since we travel more than half-time, the painting doesn't often win, but I know that the choice is mine to make.

These examples illustrate the importance of asking these questions: What do you imagine might lead to the greatest satisfaction for you? Have you given yourself the opportunity to define your interests and discover your latent talents? If the answer is yes, there is another question: Have you made a *real* commitment to the development of that skill? Are you becoming an expert? Most of us do many things adequately, or even well, but few of us have made a real commitment to the discoveries we make or the opportunities we have.

Some further thoughts about the business of settling one's own issues first. It is important to recognize that even once these questions have been answered, they don't stay answered. Circumstances change, we change, we grow, relationships change. And what makes sense for us will change, too. What is important is the quest, the search, the seizure of opportunity and refusing to accept no for an answer. Driving this quest is the conviction that there are other kinds of activities as fulfilling, as significant, and as rewarding as homemaking and mothering was at an earlier age.

The second tough task is opening the dialogue. Why is it so difficult? Not because each of us is married to an unthinking, heartless man who is unable to understand what we are struggling with. But because, however sensitive or kind or concerned he may be, he has another agenda: his practice, his own life, his own crises.

So how should a wife approach the subject?

First: She must talk about how she feels. No one can argue with you about how *you* feel. While avoiding the tendency to blame him and the easy implication that it is all somehow his fault and his responsibility, she must learn to talk about what she needs and why, not what she wants him to give or do.

Second: She should invite his reactions and suggestions early—while she is working on the task, not after she has the answer and only needs his agreement. There is a risk. He may not understand. He may see change as change for the worse, or a sign that she loves him less. But she must insist.

Third: She must not assume that he will understand without her having to say a word. This tendency to expect mind reading from the spouse is a source of enormous misunderstanding and frustration. This is another way of describing the need for the courage to confront the issues. Too many couples suffer in silence. Too many of us prefer the short-run benefits of peace at any price to the cost of long-run consequences. A creative compromise is impossible without efforts to bring these issues to the surface.

Last: Persist! Bucking the inertia of habit, the constraints of social expectations, the risks of confrontation, and the potential criticism of one's family is hard, tiring work. But the result is worth it: an unequalled opportunity for growth and development that makes possible a continuing vitality and zest for living.

—6—

Psychological Issues for the Woman Physician

Malkah T. Notman, M.D.
Carol C. Nadelson, M.D.

In the past two decades, the number of women in medical training has increased from less than 10 percent to almost 40 percent of each medical school class (Bernstein 1977). It has become acceptable, even expected, for women to enter medicine. That choice is no longer regarded as "deviant" or "masculine." But changes have been uneven, and there are still limitations and constraints on women in medicine.

According to a 1981 report from the American Association of Medical Colleges, the percentage of women actually practicing medicine has so far risen only to 10 to 11 percent from 6 percent in 1970. This reflects changes in medical school admission policies beginning in the mid-1970s. As more women enter medical practice, the social environment for them will change further, but the problems of balancing career and family responsibilities remain and are particularly difficult because of the structure of medical training and the inflexible time demands of the physician's work.

Women now in midlife and midcareer are entering their peak practice years and may also be at the midlife point in their marriages. They grew up and were trained in an era when it required a high level of interest and conviction for a woman to enter a field where prevailing patterns of training, expectations, and practice had been set by men. The choice exposed them to questions about their "femininity." For some of these women, all that was a challenge and a stimulus to competition. The structure of medical training and practice, which hardly accommodates the family and personal needs of male physicians, was even less suited to women's lives and needs.

At that time women were unwelcome in some settings, not treated as equal, and symbolically or actually not given their own "space" as colleagues. There were minor problems, such as the lack of changing or on-call rooms for women in hospitals, and more serious ones, such as a limited choice of residency programs and opportunities for practice. For example, almost no residencies in surgical specialties were open to women before the 1960s. The fact that women did not choose surgery is frequently cited as a reason, but it is difficult to choose a field perceived as closed and hostile. To go back even further, it is relevant to note that the first American medical school, founded in Philadelphia in 1765, excluded women entirely. In 1847, when Elizabeth Blackwell became the first woman to graduate from a "regular" medical school in the United States, the New York State Medical Association promptly censured the school (Nadelson 1983). In 1846, Harriet Hunt, who had established herself in an "irregular" practice in Boston, applied for admission to Harvard Medical School. She was first admitted, then rejected. It was not until 1946 that Harvard Medical School first admitted women.

Medicine as a profession is now undergoing profound changes in structure and economics. Health maintenance organizations (HMOs) have provided more salaried positions; women have generally worked in organized care settings and in salaried positions more often than men, but their pattern may soon become more like men's. Many group practices now specify that a woman should be on the staff. This makes women feel more valued, but patterns of relating to women physicians change more slowly. We will consider both the psychological characteristics of women physicians and the stresses of training and practice as they affect the woman who enters medicine.

Psychological Characteristics of Women Physicians

We do not yet have a reliable picture of women as compared to men physicians. For some years, the data measuring individual characteristics and comparing various traits of men and women, such as competence, persistence, and aggression, showed apparent and often contradictory differences. The total population available for study has been too small. Studies differed in design and assessed different attributes and were not often longitudinal or contextual. The meaning of specific findings was not at all clear, nor was the possibility considered that these measures could change with the environment.

Cartwright (1972a, 1972b, 1972c) found that female medical students differed from "traditional" women in their emphasis on individuation, self-discovery, self-expression, and self-differentiation in work. Fruen et al. (1974) found that male medical school applicants scored higher than women in dominance, exhibitionism, and order. Women had higher scores on harm avoidance, impulsivity, nurturance, understanding, and need for change. Men and women applicants did not differ in aggression, autonomy, endurance, and affiliative traits, although these traits did distinguish men and women undergraduates (Horner 1972).

McGrath and Zimet (1976) contradicted some of these findings. They found female medical students were higher on self-confidence, autonomy, and aggression than males, whereas males were higher on nurturance, affiliation, and deference. The authors attribute the results to increased numbers of women in medicine and the women's movement's support of assertiveness and non-traditional career choices.

Other studies (Notman et al. 1984) found that women medical students are fundamentally similar to other women, although very high in achievement, competence, and work orientation. They do share with other women some well-studied personality features: a tendency to be more affiliative than men, more ready to express emotion, acknowledge distress and physical symptoms, and use health care facilities. They are responsive to the opinions of others, they tend to see things in context, and they tend to negotiate and seek compromises. Gilligan (1982) described the differences in moral reasoning. Women view moral development as involving the understanding of responsibility and relationships. Men, on the other hand, see moral development as related to fairness and the understanding of rights and rules.

Differences between male and female physicians interact with the conditions of medical training and practice. The traditionally "feminine" gender role was incompatible with the qualities formerly considered important in the selection of students for medicine (Cartwright 1972a, 1972b, 1972c; Duki 1971; Epstein 1975; Fruen et al. 1974; Kimball 1973; Kosa and Coker 1965; Lopate 1968; Notman and Nadelson 1973, 1984). There is also a gender difference in the balance between nurturant and achievement wishes. Medicine has allowed men to express the need to provide caretaking and nurturance, without defeating achievement needs or compromising "masculine" goals. The situation has been different for women. Nurturant qualities have been considered "feminine," but medicine has been seen as an achievement-oriented and therefore "masculine" field. Thus women have recurrent conflicts between achievement and nurturant goals (Notman et al. 1978).

The assertiveness, competitiveness, and independence that are supported in men run counter to traditional feminine values and the socialization of women. There are important gender differences in the development of aggression and independence. The debate about gender differences in "innate" aggression (Maccoby and Jacklin 1974) is unresolved, but the developmental process in women clearly exerts a profound effect on aggression, assertiveness, and their derivatives such as competence and mastery. Girls identify with their mothers who have often internalized ideals of service and "doing for" others. For many years, medicine has been one way for a woman to attain high achievement and recognition and at the same time fulfill feminine values of care and nurturance.

The defense against sadism described by Gabbard and Menninger in Chapter 3 is more pervasive in women. The prohibitions against direct expression of aggression are more consistently part of feminine style. Awareness of being aggressive makes both men and women feel guilty and lose self-esteem, as Bibring (1953) pointed out in his discussion of the mechanism of depression. But an openly aggressive woman is also in conflict with an additional part of her ego ideal, that of femininity.

Both men and women physicians share the compulsive triad of doubt, guilt feelings, and an exaggerated sense of responsibility (Gabbard 1985), and the tendency to employ reaction formation as a defense against aggression. However, women physicians are different in some important ways. They value intimacy and attachments more and are more vulnerable to their loss; they are more expressive; they also tend more toward conformity. The woman physician often exhibits a "good girl syndrome" from having had to "do things right." In their desire for acceptance, women will accommodate to an existing style of medical behavior. This will become less constricting as a range of adaptive styles for women in medicine becomes more available and acceptable.

It is important to stress that women as well as men with a wide range of personality styles choose medicine. Some women have a more hysterical personality, although their compulsive defenses are strong enough to get them through medical school.

Women medical students and physicians may project or externalize their conflicts about activity and aggression, paying more attention to the criticisms—such as of superiors, colleagues, family—than to their own inner feelings. These conflicts can interfere with medical performance and also affect the choice of specialty and practice setting. Some women choose less difficult goals or residencies they judge to be less competitive in order to assure acceptance. This is especially true if they are married to physicians.

Women are usually the accommodators who are sensitive to the opinions of others. They tend to assume that if something does not go well, it is their fault. If there are conflicting priorities or needs, a woman readily feels guilty and responsible for the problem. This influences judgments about patient care; for example, a 1977 National Ambulatory Care Survey found that women spend more time with their patients than men do.

A woman is not only more sensitive to feelings of rejection and "dependency" but often more open about these feelings than a man might be, giving a false impression of insecurity and lack of knowledge. Concerns about separation can lead to guilt and loss of confidence. When the woman physician must choose between caring for a patient, being with her family, and tending to her own needs, she may see herself as neglectful or unable to give adequate care rather than simply making choices.

As we noted, women are more expressive than men and therefore are more likely to report symptoms and distress (Weissman and Klerman 1977). They are also more ready than men to consider seeking help and less likely to see this as incompatible with strength and competence. This may make them appear more vulnerable than they are.

Intellectual and obsessional defenses are supported by medical training, as Gabbard and Menninger describe in Chapter 3. These defenses are more prevalent in men and consistent with male personality styles. To cope with illness and death, all physicians must use distancing mechanisms that exact a price in intimacy and responsiveness. Drs. Gabbard and Menninger have discussed the differences between physicians and their spouses in the need for intimacy. In large part, these are probably male–female differences as well. Women physicians need closeness more and feel stressed if time pressures interfere with relationships. Women are not so fully sustained as men by the approval of mentors or the pursuit of perfection. They too want mastery and want to serve and rescue others; but the isolation of work undermines a particularly vital part of life for them by impairing self-esteem and nurturance provided by personal relationships. One resident, finishing a psychiatry residency said, "The only thing I really know how to do well after the past few years is to work." Pollak and Gilligan (1982), analyzing Thematic Apperception Test responses of male and female students, found that men associate danger with intimacy, and women associate it with achievement and isolation due to competitive success. They observed that medical education and practice reinforce men's fears about intimacy, because the structures and ethical codes of medicine as a profession shelter physicians from intimacy but pay little attention to the isolation it entails. The current emphasis that equates "productivity" with numbers of patients seen is likely to increase this isolationism. The impersonal care provided in many practice settings, such as HMOs, is also detrimental to intimacy.

Stresses for Women Physicians

In many ways, medical training and practice are more stressful for women than for men. We will consider the following sources of stress particular to women: (1) minority status; (2) life stage considerations; (3) isolation; (4) social role conflict; (5) singlehood; and (6) pregnancy.

Phelps (1968), before the recent increase in numbers of women physicians, reported that dropout rates from medical school for academic reasons were similar for male and female students. However, of those leaving for nonacademic reasons (usually personal), 8 percent were females and 3 percent were males. This gap is closing; the difference in attrition between male and female medical students is now vanishing.

Adsett (1968) reported that a greater percentage of women medical students than men sought psychiatric counseling. He commented that this might be due simply to women's greater propensity to ask for help. Women in the United States generally use psychiatric facilities more than do men (Gove and Tudor 1973). Weinberg and Rooney (1973) cited "problems of adjustment," related to the small numbers of women in medical school, as a source of their lower academic achievement. Performance differences no longer exist.

Minority Status

Many of women's difficulties in medicine were due to their minority status and the accompanying prejudice, discrimination, and scapegoating. They still have not reached positions of leadership. In 1987 there were only two women deans of United States medical schools and few chairs of departments in schools and hospitals. The young woman physician has few role models, and the middle-aged woman physician had even fewer. The networks of communication and support still have many "old boy" aspects. Subtle exclusion persists. Women still phrase comments tentatively, as compared to the greater directness of men; they are less often heard in meetings and are more likely to be overlooked in promotions and selection for prominent positions.

Although women physicians are gradually appearing in more advertisements, the female pronoun is rarely used in referring to "the doctor"; it will take some time before women are fully integrated into the profession.

When women perceived that they were not included, or were the objects of criticism, sarcasm, or sexual joking, they tended to feel that they were at fault and withdrew. If they were to respond with overt hostility, that could be interpreted as a fitting response to the mobilization of forbidden ambitions or aggressive strivings—a punishment for "daring" and competing, and a confirmation that they did not belong.

What we have come to understand in this past decade, documented by studies of a wide range of developmental, educational, and work situations, is the extent to which male cognitive and achievement styles have structured socialization, teaching, and rewards, and have contributed to women's feeling of being at odds, being second best, and not being truly "right" in that context (Gilligan 1982; Hall and Sandler 1982). Such feelings clearly affect personal comfort, self-esteem, and relationships, including marriages.

Life Stage Considerations

Although graduate training and careers have now been accepted as part of legitimate aspirations for women, working out the life course patterns has not been so clear. As Perun and Del Vento Bielby (1981) pointed out, the work trajectory and the family trajectory of women are simultaneous in many cases, and much of this congruence is new. Knowledge and support are unevenly available. Some peers are marrying and having families, although training demands make it difficult. Sayres et al. (1986) documented the difficulty faced by pregnant women in training in the Harvard teaching hospitals. Women who do not have families often feel "out of synch" with peers, doubting their femininity and their competence in areas other than work. Women who do not have partners often find the work demands to be isolating. Many conceal their occupations when dating, because some men are still intimidated by intellectually accomplished women. A woman physician who has children relatively late may feel "abnormal." The problem is most serious in geographical regions and social groups where professional women are uncommon.

Self-concepts of being "old" or "young," appropriate or outdated, "right" or "wrong," reflect both social norms and internal processes. Little is known in this area. Ideas about "normality" need changing to reflect current social realities. Judgments about one's normality and assessments of where one fits influence self-esteem; feelings of being "out of synch" with what is expected influences the sense of normality (Neugarten 1968).

Women's career and family patterns have changed a good deal in the last two decades. There is more freedom for undertaking childbearing after age 25 because of better health, improved technology, and more obstetrical experience. Yet women carry with them concepts of how to live as a woman, which are derived from identifications with an older generation of mothers and grandmothers. Thus women may find their new lives confusing or unsatisfying, especially if there are few supports and models. Becoming a parent at an age when a career has already shaped a woman's self-definition presents different combinations of strengths and vulnerabilities than those of the young physician mother who is simultaneously exploring both worlds.

Isolation

Isolation can be literal or emotional. Training and residency can be isolating in both ways for both men and women. Work leaves little time for the development of relationships and personal priorities. Meanwhile, there is pressure to work for personal fulfillment, rather than social or communal welfare. These pressures affect women and men differently because of their different personality styles and needs.

Once in practice, physicians may suffer from their earlier lack of attention to sustaining relationships. Alcohol and drug use are one result. Mood disorders and suicide are more common in women than men physicians (Steppacher and Mausner 1974), partly because of loneliness and partly due to role strain.

Another kind of isolation is geographic. A woman physician may be sent to a remote spot to fulfill service obligations, because an opening is available or because a leadership position is available. Once there, she may find it difficult to make social contacts. Often she has no real peers—few or no professional women—or no one comfortable with her socially. Women in leadership roles in many fields say it is hard to find someone with whom they can "let down their hair" without risking loss of face and social status. Some women, however, can tolerate this kind of isolation better, or have close friends or family elsewhere, or are particularly skillful at breaking down barriers.

> Dr. Betty was a senior faculty member in a department of pediatrics. She had become a professor after many years at teaching, research, and work in various administrative positions in both the university department and the hospital. Shortly after she was appointed to a major administrative position, she found herself feeling very lonely. She was sought after by women for help in their promotions and criticized by them when they were disappointed. She found few people to whom she could talk freely about the problems in the department. Male members of the department were resentful of her prominence. In effect, she was regarded as the department "mother," not departmental chair, and asked to solve problems more appropriate to a parent than to a director. The stress became so great that she left to take another position.

Social Role Conflict

Despite the feminization of work, career, and working, women retain their social roles as the household managers and primary caretakers of children and elderly parents. Most professional women use substitute care for which they assume major responsibility. In a survey of Harvard Medical School alumni 10 years after graduation, only one woman reported that her husband took care of their young child (Nadelson et al. 1979).

Some physician fathers have become more involved in their families, but usually the woman experiences more conflicts of priorities. The woman feels she is confronted by unfulfillable demands, and this creates tension about loyalties and commitments. Most women find ways to reconcile the conflict; but the woman who is perfectionistic, compulsive, or has ambivalent or guilty relationships with people she is trying to please may have particular difficulties.

Marriage itself causes more stress for women than for men (Bernard 1973; Gove and Tudor 1973). On the other hand, working women have better mental health (Baruch et al. 1983). The married career woman does not suffer the homemaker's loss of status and diversity in experience nor the resulting damage to self-esteem. However, she is still often expected to modify her work patterns to spend more time at home or to be available to her husband: an external expectation she often internalizes. The role strain can be considerable.

Singlehood

In the past, career women and intellectual women usually remained childless and often unmarried. In some areas of the United States as well as in Europe and India, household servants were more readily available, and this made a medical career less difficult for a woman with a family.

Remaining single is still a choice for many women physicians because of greater mobility, more acceptance, and the ability to conduct most activities without a "protective man."

For women who seek freedom for personal development, remaining single has major advantages. It provides freedom from the conflicts and negotiations with a spouse; it offers a chance for solitude, reflection, and autonomous decision making. Self-sufficiency may be adaptive and personally rewarding.

The disadvantages of singleness have many sources. There are the problems of minority status and the anxiety of others about a relationship with a single woman. Related problems are loneliness and lack of companionship and sharing. The advantages and the problems must be carefully weighed by each woman.

A pattern now emerging more openly than ever before is a lesbian partnership. Sometimes this choice is made early, during school years, and sometimes it is made after a marriage and children. Some of these relationships are also a feminist political statement. A stereotyped view of lesbian relationships is that they are inevitably turbulent or involve excessive "dependency." Many, however, are in fact stable and mutually growth-promoting. The problems of adapting to mutual needs, dealing with competition, priorities, and allocation of work are similar to those of dual-career heterosexual couples.

Pregnancy

The physician who becomes pregnant while in training, particularly in residency, faces acute conflicts in relation to the needs of her patients and colleagues, and concern about her own health. Time demands are likely to be inflexible because her peers are intimately affected by her availability and capacity to work. It is easy to lose the sense of pregnancy as an experience to be enjoyed.

> Dr. Anna was a 30-year-old resident in her next to last year of a primary care residency program. She and her husband had planned to have a baby when she finished her residency. Her husband, a lawyer, became ill. To their relief, it turned out not to be life-threatening, but while they were preoccupied with the problem, she became pregnant. They recognized that this was not what they had planned, but also understood that it was in part an unconscious response to his illness: insuring that life would continue. Realistic concern about the pregnancy and baby now took over. Dr. Anna was able to interrupt her residency for 2 months, then return to work. But she was resented by colleagues who had had to cover for her. When she returned to work, the chief resident had made the next year's assignments: her assignment was especially demanding to make up for the lost time. Yet she was also required to return for an extra 2 months of residency.

Some women do become preoccupied with their own welfare and use the pregnancy as an excuse to avoid onerous duties, but this happens infrequently.

Pregnancy stirs strong emotions in both patients and colleagues, who can be surprisingly unsupportive. In patients it may evoke envy, disappointment, unresolved feelings about siblings, anger at parents, and sexual competitiveness with the doctor. Patients may express these feelings by becoming pregnant.

All this can be particularly stressful for the physician who is not accustomed to such variations in her own moods, feelings, and physical capacity. Institutions have been rather unaccommodating to the needs of the pregnant physician, expecting her to go on with business as usual (Sayres et al. 1986). The increasing numbers of women in medicine will undoubtedly bring changes in these attitudes.

Once the baby is born, the emotional involvement and lack of sleep make a demanding practice particularly stressful. Many women must either delegate child care or curtail their work during this period, with varying degrees of comfort or conflict. Resolution of the conflicts can be facilitated by a supportive husband who shares responsibilities. Friends not only provide support, but *also* validate the woman's choices and reduce her feelings of guilt.

Conclusion

In the 1960s and early 1970s, some believed that the growing presence of women in medicine would humanize the field. Those expecting such change may have been somewhat disappointed so far. Still, time may demonstrate changes in medical practice that make for a better fit between the psychological characteristics of women physicians and the demands of the profession.

7

The Woman Physician's Marriage

Carol C. Nadelson, M.D.
Malkah T. Notman, M.D.

Most women physicians marry, and about three-quarters of them marry physicians or other professionals. Dual-career couples in the mid-1980s are mutually interdependent, with a strong attachment to ideals of companionship, communication, and sharing as well as pursuing individual goals; but an imbalance between the partners persists. As Bernard (1973) pointed out, marriage has always required wives to make more compromises and sacrifices than their husbands; the dual-career marriage has not changed that. Even now, women often view their husbands' careers as more important than their own. When they do not, there may be strains in the marriage. These attitudes derive from many generations of socialization. Women are seen as less serious about their work than men in comparable fields. This creates a further conflict for a woman physician who is already struggling to balance her career commitment and loyalty to patients with her role in her family.

In families in which the husband is a physician and the wife is not, wives are even more likely to see themselves as playing mainly supportive roles, even if they have careers of their own. A woman physician's nonphysician husband is less likely to adopt that view of his role; if circumstances demand it, strains and difficulties may develop.

The view of men and women is more likely to be egalitarian during medical school and the early training period, but even at that stage there are differences. A recent interview study of female interns and residents and their husbands compared data with a previous study of male physicians and their wives, and found substantial differences (Kelner and Rosenthal 1986). Wives of male physicians were gratified by their husbands' fulfillment of career goals and pleased to be supportive. The husbands of women physicians found this kind of support to their wives less personally rewarding and more an onerous obligation.

In both studies, spouses were bothered by the fatigue of their partner, the lack of time together, and the need to postpone important sources of gratification. Husbands of female physicians tended to feel overburdened with domestic responsibilities that seemed to hamper their own careers. Wives of male physicians reported no such conflict, even when they were working to help finance their husbands' medical training.

Both male and female physicians and students valued emotional security and intimacy provided by marriage and were relieved about not having to date. But both groups of spouses worried about growing apart from their mates. Husbands of physicians were more concerned about the extreme narrowing of their spouses' field of interest during medical training; wives of physicians were more concerned about being outgrown by their better-educated partners. Husbands of physicians resented their situation and blamed the medical profession for the strain on their marriages; wives of physicians coped by vicarious identification with their partners' goals and by trying not to complain by keeping future rewards in mind.

Both male and female physicians complained about the demands on their time and energy and the resulting short-changing of their partners (although men worried less about this). They were also anxious about conflicting role obligations. Having children was another source of strain for the women. Most of them planned to choose a specialty that would permit them more time with the family. It is widely believed that the stress of long work hours contributes to family turmoil in the traditional marriage, but as Gabbard and Menninger have pointed out in Chapter 2, the data do not support this hypothesis.

Stress, Adaptation, and Costs

The picture of a compulsive workaholic with a dependent spouse certainly does not fit most female physicians. We will consider some of the dual-career patterns that are particularly relevant for women physicians. Many studies of dual-career marriages have reported greater stress and unhappiness for the husbands of working women. These studies, however, generally looked at non-representative samples because the data were often collected very early in the history of the dual-career phenomenon. Many of the studies were also influenced by traditional social and political values. Today it does not seem that husbands of employed wives suffer more stress than husbands of homemakers. In fact, for some men, a high-achieving employed wife is a "supermom" whose achievement offers him nurturance via her competence rather than competition.

Dual careers require organization, trust, and integration, especially when husband and wife have different career goals. Both usually expect the marriage to support high-level, energy-depleting, and sometimes emotionally intensive work. In two-physician families, the daily business of life may be "on hold," especially early in the partners' careers. Career priorities may preclude attention to personal needs.

All dual-career couples have trouble finding time to be with each other, but physician couples have special problems. One couple, both family practitioners in a small town, found that they had to take separate vacations because somebody had to cover the practice. It was several years before they worked out coverage arrangements with other local physicians—less because of their patients' needs and fears than because of their own worries about abandoning them. Physicians like to be in control, make decisions, and assume responsibility. When both partners have similar needs and personality styles, it may be difficult for either to find a respite.

Gender-Related Personality Differences

In this situation men and women place different values on their relationships and their needs for support.

The Drs. J. provide an illustration. They met in medical school, where both were top students, and married shortly afterward. Robert J. became a surgeon and Mary J. combined research with clinical practice.

When Robert's mother became seriously ill and died after several months, he was able to continue to work, although he was quite shaken by the loss. Mary was prepared to take time off to spend with him and his family. Robert was appreciative but dealt with much of his mourning by himself; he was somewhat withdrawn and abruptly threw himself back into work. Some time later, Mary developed a gynecological illness requiring a series of surgical procedures. She had always prided herself on stoicism and was reluctant to reveal her problem to anyone at work, but she counted on her husband for support. She wanted him to accompany her for her treatments, but he was reluctant to take the time. Considerable tension arose when she contrasted his attitude with hers when his mother died. This vignette indicates differences between men and women in personality and adaptive style. Women are less likely to equate unexpressiveness and rigidity with strength. Mary felt abandoned by her husband and betrayed by his loyalty to the "strong, silent" ideal.

Despite hopes, wishes, and promises of "having it all," the complexities of dual-career relationships are difficult to work out. Partners married to physicians must expect unanticipated compromises and changes. Men in our culture have not grown up expecting to have to adapt to another person's work and career ambitions. Even when they want to be "good guys" and adhere to equality, it may cause depression, conflicts about work, displaced anger, or self-defeating or passive-aggressive behavior.

Division of Labor

Women continue to bear the major responsibility for family and home, despite their career obligations. Heins et al. (1977b) studied a group of women physicians and reported that the vast majority did the housework. Married women physicians often complain that they fall asleep in the evening over journals, books, and papers, while their physician husbands seem to have renewed energy. One reason for this may be a conflict about the more academic or "ambitious" aspects of their medical work. Often they share with their husbands the expectation that the men will pursue more academic interests (Nadelson and Nadelson 1988).

The male partner is often self-congratulatory about and rewarded with accolades for any "helpfulness." Women, however, are *expected* to run the household. If they do not sail through with grace, they often consider themselves failures, and their family and friends support that conclusion. Both partners generally conclude that each needs "a good wife" (Nadelson and Nadelson 1988).

Rigid role patterns cannot survive serious career demands. These relationships require a balance of power and responsibility, with implicit or explicit guidelines and rules as well as flexibility.

The partners must implicitly trust each other; yet competition, anger, and tension about sex roles may remain active. Despite commitment, love, and respect, attitudes are historically slow to change, especially when they are only partially conscious. Even in 1988, a husband, his family, and even his friends may perceive the wife with a career as too aggressive or, with some tutoring, as "castrating." A husband must eventually come to understand that the doctor he married would not be successful if she weren't aggressive. Some marriages cannot tolerate this strain.

There are also problems when the wife tries to be accommodating and acquiescent in situations that demand decisiveness. Even the couple who enters such a marriage with their eyes open must learn to tolerate unanticipated frustration, resentment, and jealousy (Nadelson and Nadelson 1988).

Responsibility for Children

Attitudes about having children have changed. Highly educated women expect fewer children than other women. A 1983 study reported that about 20 percent of women in professional and managerial occupations, or with postgraduate education, plan to have no children (Moore et al. 1987); only 7 percent of women who never completed high school expect no children.

For dual-career couples, children bring new demands and priorities. Everyday activities require more coordination. In an emergency, concern for the children must take priority over other obligations. When a child is ill or needs extra attention, most husbands assume that the wife will take care of the matter. This shift toward traditional roles comes as a surprise to many couples who consider themselves liberated and egalitarian (Gaddy et al. 1983; Nadelson and Nadelson 1988). The wives feel pressed to be both supermoms and superphysicians. Children's schools, other professionals, and service providers generally assume that there is always a "wife" at home who has no other commitments. This presents problems for the physician mother unless she has comprehensive substitute care. Nine-to-five day care alone is hardly sufficient, given a physician's schedule. Women who remain employed while rearing young children, however, are more likely to rise in the profession (Weitzman 1985).

Now, however, there is evidence of change. A young man recently became president of Future Homemakers of America. Many men now assume that they will take a major role in child rearing, and they are making the necessary career changes. But the role change creates problems for them. Osherson and Dill (1983) (whose studies did not include many physicians) found that egalitarian husbands felt that they were less successful at work, although they had more career flexibility and more room for self-development.

Men in dual-career couples work more hours than women; both men and women in higher prestige occupations work more hours than those of the same sex in less prestigious occupations. Both men and women work long hours when their spouses do. In general, when occupational status is high, there is greater equality of occupational involvement.

After children are grown up, some formerly successful adaptations show strains. Women have more varied career trajectories and timetables than men. The following vignette illustrates some of these dilemmas:

> Drs. K. married when Jane K. was a resident and Arthur K., 10 years older, was establishing an active medical career. They chose to remain in the city where they trained and could both work. They had two children. Jane continued to practice as a member of a group with steady hours and a predictable income, while Arthur became head of a university department. As he reached his mid-60s and faced a change in administration, he wanted to retire and take a senior teaching post offered to him in another state, where he could reduce his professional activity while retaining his status. But Jane had recently left the group practice for a position she enjoyed greatly; she was unenthusiastic about moving. During this time, Arthur became depressed. He felt isolated and uncared for. His dependency needs were not met by his wife as her activity increased and his diminished. She was caught between her wish to be caring and her wish to pursue new opportunities.

Income Discrepancies

Another problem confronting women physicians is financial. On the average, male physicians earn 30 percent more per hour than female physicians (Salsberger et al. 1987). Generally, the income differential decreases as years of work increase (Nadelson and Nadelson 1988). This situation, however, creates special problems for many young women physicians. They have financial problems as they struggle to pay off training debts, liability insurance, and practice overhead, especially if they must work fewer hours because of child-rearing responsibilities.

In this chapter, we are distinguishing between dual-career and dual-worker families. More than 50 percent of American families now include at least two working adults, but "dual career" implies a commitment to professions that involve a workweek longer than 40 hours. Twenty percent of U.S. couples live in dual-career families; husbands usually earn more than their wives and have more prestigious positions. Some men like having their caretaking women earn more money, but many are uneasy when their wives earn more than they do, especially in a male-dominated field like medicine.

When the woman physician is more successful than her husband, there are special pressures for both partners. The woman may unconsciously compensate by sabotaging her own success, or by developing physical or psychiatric symptoms.

> Linda F., age 50, was married to a lawyer, James F., age 53. He was in a middle-level position in his law firm and expected no further advances. While their children were growing up, she worked in emergency medicine. After they left home, she took advantage of the flexible hours permitted by a residency in psychiatry. She was exceedingly successful, but became very anxious when she realized that she was outstripping her husband professionally. Her anxiety became so great that she sought psychotherapy.

The emerging health care delivery system provides greater numbers of salaried jobs with fixed schedules—an advantage to women physicians with small children. But the costs of medical school and liability insurance have also been growing. Many women physicians find themselves unable to repay debts or keep up with malpractice premiums.

Geographic Mobility

Another problem of dual-career couples is the geographic mobility necessary for career advances. Wives and husbands still differ in their willingness to follow a spouse to another city. One study reported that 68 percent of wives were reluctant to consider a position in another city unless their husbands also had an offer; 40 percent of the husbands would consider moving in the same situation. A 1982 study (Kilpatrick 1982) reported that 35 percent of male candidates who were finalists for positions requiring relocation would not negotiate further unless their wives' needs were also met. This may contribute to women's problems in making career progress.

One solution is the commuter marriage, in which partners live in different cities and see each other mainly on weekends and holidays. Less than 1 percent of dual-career couples in the United States (about 1 million) live a commuter life. It seems to be rare among physicians because medical schedules are so demanding.

Midlife Stresses

There are several critical points in medical marriages: (*1*) establishment of the relationship and exploration of roles and work patterns; (*2*) the arrival of children and the need for new adaptations; and (*3*) the completion of child rearing, which allows the wife to shift her priorities toward work.

When physician couples are at midcareer and midlife, the wife is usually in a general practice and the husband is in a specialty; or the wife is working in an organized medical care setting and the husband is in a demanding academic hierarchy. A difficult shift in expectations occurs if the wife decides to try to change her career or return to previously relinquished goals.

> The Drs. L. illustrate another pattern. Martha L., a psychiatrist, practiced from an office in her home, while her husband, John L., developed a research career and became increasingly successful academically. When the children left home, Martha felt increasingly angry, isolated, and resentful of her husband for not supporting her career.

Women physicians are also expected to serve as primary caretakers during the illness of a parent, in-law, or husband.

> The Drs. M. were both internists in their mid-30s, successful researchers with bright futures. Fred M. developed bipolar affective disorder and was hospitalized. Virginia M. became angry and resentful, unable to adapt to the increased burden of his illness while caring for the children. His vulnerability was particularly difficult for her, as it is for many physicians.

Illness represents failure for those seeking to control their lives and health; adaptation to it becomes particularly difficult.

Another circumstance causing stress for women physicians is the retirement of an older husband.

Mr. N. was a 63-year-old recently retired art dealer; Dr. N. was a 50-year-old hospital administrator. They sought therapy because of Mr. N.'s depression. He had been highly successful but was forced to retire early when his business began to fail because of increased competition. He expected to use the time he had to write and travel, but he had not anticipated the change in the direction of his wife's career. Dr. N. had worked part time in outpatient clinics while the children were growing up. When they went away to college, she began to take on more responsibility at the hospital where she worked. When Mr. N. retired, Dr. N. discovered that they had less money than she had thought, so she accepted a full-time position. Mr. N. found her increasingly more distant and unmindful of his needs.

Divorce

Social commentators who see dark days ahead cite rising divorce rates. Present reality is compared with a romanticized past in which families supposedly stayed together and divorce was rare. We must, however, place this in perspective. Increased longevity means that a marriage will now last through what used to be two lifetimes. Less than a century ago, death in childbirth, occupational hazards, and infections limited the number of adults who reached middle and old age. Marriages often lasted little more than a decade before the death of one partner. The "decay of the American family" has become a greater concern only when divorce (rather than death) dissolves the partnership and causes "abandonment" of children. Nevertheless, as many as 60 percent of marriages today will last until the death of one partner.

Divorce rates are said to be higher in dual-career couples, although it is difficult to assess these reports accurately. Divorce is three times as likely among women earning more than $15,000 per year as it is among women earning less than $3,000 a year. For every $1,000 increase in the wife's earnings, the divorce rate rises by 2 percent (Johnson 1981). Hiller and Philliber (1982) suggested that wives who exceed the achievements of their husbands are at higher risk for divorce or negative job change. Social commentators with a more optimistic outlook, and who are more comfortable with social change, do not find these statistics so upsetting. Women who earn a higher salary have more freedom to leave an unrewarding marriage.

Conclusion

Stereotyped attitudes about women who achieve persist. Head-lines still say "Grandmother Receives Nobel Prize" (referring to scientist Rosalyn Yalow) or "Mother of Two Heads Psychiatrists" (referring to the first author of this chapter being elected president of the American Psychiatric Association). Motherhood is still seen as the marker of "normality" for women, although the view is now less openly expressed. Attitudinal change is slow. As a woman physician recently commented, men accept women as profession-als, but they're not ready to accept them as true peers (Jones 1987). It is the same at home. We look toward a future in which married men and women physicians can join in a partnership as peers and colleagues at home as well as at work.

8

Sexual Problems in Physician Couples

Domeena C. Renshaw, M.D.

"The Lonely Life of an Ob-Gyn Doctor's Wife" was the headline of an Ann Landers column (*Chicago Sun-Times*, August 18, 1985). Good-naturedly and humorously, the wife wrote of wishing that her husband would spend more time at home. Meals and family events were rarely shared since patients took precedence. "Exhaustion is another problem. I can't count the number of times my darling has fallen asleep in the middle of a conversation, or worse yet, while making love—or trying to. . . ." It was signed "Dedicated Wife of a Dedicated M.D."

Most physicians would agree that exhaustion is an occupational stress for them. Batches of 24-hour shifts are routine. However, one study of physician marriages showed no correlation between long hours and dissatisfaction or divorce (Garvey and Tuason 1979). In the survey by Gabbard et al. described in Chapter 2, those who worked longer hours did not even have sexual relations less often. In this same survey, physician couples who had sought marital counseling spent an average of only 37.8 minutes a day talking with each other, although sexual contact averaged 1.4 times per week. One wonders how long dentists or lawyers and their spouses talk to each other.

Doctors' sex lives have filled the pages of novels, magazines, film scripts, and television soap operas for many years. The doctor hero is usually strong and sexy—"tall, lean, rugged, with a square jaw and steel-gray eyes." Recently, blond, bright, beautiful, young, slim female doctors have been featured. How accurate are these images? Quincy, with his string of glamorous dates, is hardly typical. Nor is the suave and elegant family doctor Marcus Welby, who offers coffee to adoring young nurses. Handsome Ben Casey saved children's lives in each episode and enjoyed the breathless gratitude of gorgeous long-lashed young mothers. The public clearly wants to watch doctors romancing. Young girls still dream of a doctor husband, and mercenary parents may scheme and plan such a marriage for their daughters.

Women doctors have special problems here. As their education and income rise, they have fewer potential partners. A woman doctor is far more intimidating to a less educated man than a male doctor is to a less educated woman. Men are still expected to show dominance and control in marriage, and many women doctors strain to appear "traditional." They may act inferior and helpless at home in an attempt to bolster the self-esteem of a younger, less educated, less adequate, or lower-earning mate. A few use their superior knowledge as a put-down, increasing the danger of divorce.

Malpractice suits, consumer power, civil rights, freedom of information, "third-party payer power," peer review, and physician self-studies have all paved the way for the fine art of lampooning doctors in bold newspaper headlines: "Even many docs see sex as a hazard to health" (Detroit), or "Doctors rate so-so in sex guidance" (Chicago). Reporter Jon Van was astounded at the findings of a 1979 American Academy of Family Practice (AAFP) life-style study comparing the sexuality views of executives, doctors, farmers, secretaries, teachers, and garment workers. The question was: "Do you feel any of the following practices can be physically harmful? Masturbation/Intercourse/Oral Sex/Homosexual Practice/Extramarital Sex/Group Sex?" The results indicated that "doctors appeared to know less about sex than farmers and secretaries." They said masturbation and oral sex were harmful.

Soon after the Van article came Cynthia Smith's (1980) survey of unhappy doctors' wives. Smith, an editor-publisher of *Medical Magazine*, reported that many of these wives said their husbands were oafish, inexperienced lovers who drove them into depressed, angry, and unhappy patienthood. "Only by being a patient can the doctor's family get his attention, and then he only gives orders." The book was given full-page newspaper coverage, and numerous magazine articles advised women not to marry doctors because they were "lousy lovers."

Spoofs followed, including *101 Ways Not to Have Sex Tonight* by I. M. Potent, M.D., and *The Joy of No Sex*. Of the 101 excuses given by Dr. I. M. Potent for avoiding sex at home, the one that gets the strongest reaction is: "I already gave at the office." This touches, of course, on the concern of the physician's wife about attractive young nurses, technicians, volunteers, secretaries, and patients.

When I see one of my male peers come down the corridor 40 pounds lighter with Grecian Formula on his hair and wearing a Gucci outfit, I wonder whether his wife will soon be in my office because he is requesting a divorce. When she comes she will usually say that they have had no sex for several months: "He was always too tired." Often she asks about "midlife crisis" and "male menopause." These popular generalizations should not replace individual evaluation of the marital relationship. A man or a woman physician may use an affair to ward off concerns about normal aging or self-worth. At times it is a misguided search for self-help sex therapy when a partner is blamed for a sexual symptom. For some it represents rejuvenation, reaffirmation of self-esteem, or "not missing out," the same rationalizations used by nonphysicians. When there is or was an affair, the most common sexual symptom in the marriage is inhibited sexual desire (ISD).

Traditional physician marriages in the United States often start with an attractive wife who works to help her tired, impecunious medical student husband. Later the balance may change: a desirable male physician who attracts available females in the health care system. The doctor's wife becomes concerned when sex is "number 24" on the daily "to do" list, and he is spending long evening hours at the hospital, or when there are phone calls in a female voice that sounds a little too familiar. Suspicions become worries, then questions, then accusations. Fights and demands ensue: "Tell me you love me!" "Make love to me right now!" "It's me or medicine!" The wife may seek a lover herself. Revenge or solace? Love or an "ego trip"? At this point, one of them may seek help.

Both male and female physicians may be "bigamously" married to medicine (Garvey and Tuason 1979; Glick and Borus 1984; Wolf 1978). Female physicians must also fulfill the demanding role of wife and mother, and they often struggle needlessly with guilt about their children's problems, even though those problems may be unrelated to their medical careers (Anonymous 1985).

The woman doctor does not have more hired help than nonphysician peers. She feels she must shop, remember social engagements, and attend PTA meetings more regularly than her male colleagues. Hospitals often ignore this; one director of residency education, when I complained that I had not had time to complete a reading assignment, told me that, "No one asked you to do medicine. You have to keep up or else!"

The woman physician needs an extra gift of tact and sensitivity when her income exceeds that of her spouse. She must ensure that his worth is not measured in dollars in their own relationship. She may also hesitate to initiate sex for fear of undercutting a male prerogative. Just as a male physician's wife needs to develop self-esteem and success for her own fulfillment and enjoyment, so must the husband of a woman doctor evolve an autonomous sense of worth and satisfaction.

There is little information about the incidence of sexual dysfunctions, either in the general population or in physicians. One study of 100 "normal" couples reported that almost half of them had sexual problems (Frank et al. 1978). Since sex clinics see only those with problems, it is uncertain how many medical marriages have satisfactory sexual relations. But it is alarming how often physicians resort to unproven and potentially harmful solutions to their sexual problems. A special risk is the use of experimentally self-administered "erection therapy." Some examples I have observed are: (*1*) self-administered testosterone injections, which increased libido without producing an erection; (*2*) nitroglycerine ointment applied at the base of the penis, which "burnt my wife's vagina for days"; (*3*) ingestion of yohimbine over a 3-month period, which "only made me nervous, but I couldn't tolerate more than 15 mg a day"; (*4*) vasopressin nasal spray, which "gave me a better orgasm, but did nothing for my erections"; and (*5*) injections of papaverine, which "sometimes helps me get an erection—but why do they sometimes fail?" None of these physicians had had an impotence workup. Why do well-educated medical men take such needless risks, when reading available sex manuals and applying extended loveplay could do so much more to enhance their relationships?

Profile of Sample Presented

Of the 953 couples treated in 13½ years at the Loyola Sexual Dysfunction Training Clinic (abbreviated hereafter as "Clinic"), 36 (4 percent) have included physicians. The program at Loyola is a 7-week (35 hours) training clinic with therapists of both sexes.

In addition to these couples, I have treated 77 (20 female) solo physicians as a private practitioner. These include 9 male and 2 female residents, as well as 10 male and 4 female medical students. With them I performed modified sex therapy in two to eight 1-hour visits after a 2-hour evaluation.

A cross section of the sexual symptoms of the 1,906 patients treated at the Clinic is presented in Table 1.

It is worthwhile to compare our sample of 113 physicians with other professional groups, such as attorneys, dentists, veterinarians, psychologists, and social workers (Table 2).

Physicians' symptoms were similar to those of other professionals (Table 3).

Physician and medical student ages ranged from 25 to 66 years. Forty-one of the physician couple patients were Catholic; 30 were Jewish; 28 Protestant; 2 Hindu; 2 Moslem; and 10 had no religious affiliation. This religious breakdown was similar to that of the total Clinic population (TP). Only half of the TP practiced their religion regularly. Nonpracticing as well as church-attending professionals admitted inhibitions and guilt about masturbation and oral sex. Medical specialties included internist, orthopedic surgeon, general surgeon, gynecologist, pathologist, thoracic surgeon, radiologist, pediatrician, dermatologist, family practitioner, chiropractor, and psychiatrist. Endocrinology fellows, residents, and medical students also participated.

Table 1. Profile of 953 Couples at Loyola Sex Clinic, July 1972–December 1985

Sexual Diagnosis	N	Male	Female
Inhibited sexual desire	522	225	297
Inhibited female orgasm	513	. . .	513
Inhibited male orgasm (impotence)	356	356	. . .
Premature ejaculation	165	165	. . .
Premature ejaculation and impotence	67	67	. . .
Functional dyspareunia	43	2	41
Functional vaginismus	58	. . .	58
Unconsummated marriage	58	. . .	. . .
Zero sexual symptom	182	89	93

Note. N = 1,906 (total population).

Table 2. Comparative Profile of "Professionals" Seeking Sex Therapy, Loyola University Medical Center, 1972–1985

	No. of Couples	Male: Sexual Symptoms		Female: Sexual Symptoms		Alcohol Abuse, Past		Alcohol Abuse, Current		Affair, Past		Affair, Current		Previous Marriages	
		Present	Absent	Present	Absent	M	F	M	F	M	F	M	F	M	F
MD	36	24	6	3	3	11	1	3	0	10	1	2	1	6	0
Spouse	36	3	3	16	8	3	0	1	2	1	8	1	1	3	4
Solo MD (postgrad)	…	38	…	14	…	3	…	0	…	6	…	0	…	26	4
Solo resident	…	9	…	2	…	0	…	0	…	…	…	…	…	1	0
Solo medical student	…	10	…	4	…	0	…	0	…	…	…	…	…	0	0
Dentist	26	22	4	…	…	4	0	2	0	8	0	2	0	1	0
Spouse	26	0	0	14	8	0	1	0	2	0	4	0	2	0	0
Veterinarian	3	3	…	…	…	0	0	0	0	3	0	1	0	0	0
Spouse	3	…	…	1	2	0	0	0	0	0	0	0	0	0	0
Attorney	68	45	11	10	2	7	1	1	1	27	4	4	1	11	2
Spouse	68	8	4	30	26	2	1	1	0	2	8	1	1	5	1
Social Worker/ Psychologist	33	24	0	6	3	1	0	0	0	6	2	2	2	1	1
Spouse	33	5	4	14	10	0	1	0	0	2	1	2	1	1	1

Note. The total population consisted of 409 persons: 243 professionals and 166 spouses, 113 MDs (77 solo MDs + 36 as couples), and 116 as couples in 7-week Clinic (mixed professionals).

Table 3. Comparative Sexual Symptom Profile

	Dentist (N=26)		Attorney (N=68)		Social Worker/ Psychologist (N=33)		MD (N=113)	
	N	%	N	%	N	%	N	%
Impotence	7	27	21	31	10	30	30	26
Premature ejaculation	14	54	10	15	10	30	31	27
Inhibited sexual desire (male)	1	4	14	21	4	12	22	19
Inhibited sexual desire (female)	...		5	7	3	9	10	9
Anorgasmia	...		4	6	3	9	11	10
Vaginismus	...		1	1	...		...	
No sexual symptom (male)	4	15	11	16	...		6	5
No sexual symptom (female)	...		2	3	3	9	3	3
Unconsummated marriage in the above	...		1	1	...		2	2

The 7-week sex treatment program is the clinical segment of a 10-week elective training rotation for trainees who work in the Clinic. They are given 15 hours (3 weeks) of didactic workshops and then 35 hours (7 weeks) of structured couples treatment by the dual-sex trainee team. I provide direct on-site supervision, along with several co-supervisors who are apprentices. Usually more than 100 couples are on our waiting list; the wait is 4 to 14 months.

Each of the seven Clinic sessions lasts 5 hours, beginning and ending with a roundtable discussion between the patient couple and the dual-sex team. During these discussions, the participants examine the past week's events of home and the evening's tasks; they are then debriefed before they leave. In each session they look inward at the self, backward at the past, and outward at the relationship. Each partner fills in questionnaires; feedback on the questionnaires is given in weeks 5, 6, and 7. Week 1 is for history-taking: personal, medical, and sexual. Week 2 includes audiovisual aids for explicit sex education: anatomy, physiology, timing differences between male and female responses, myths, medication effects, dysfunctions, and treatment techniques to be practiced at home (Renshaw 1983).

In week 2 each patient is also given a thorough physical examination and a sexological examination in the presence of the

Figure 1. A Loyola Therapist's Final Evaluation Upon Completion of Sex Therapy (one for each partner).

Patient's Name: _____   Therapist's Name: _____

Date: _____

1. Sex problem on starting program: _____

2. Sex problem now: worse/same/somewhat improved/much improved/better

3. Therapist's prediction for their sex problem 6 months from today:
   worse/same/somewhat improved/much improved/better

4. Therapist's comparison (circle one)

	8 Weeks Ago	Now
a) nudity in bed	never/sometimes/often	never/sometimes/often
b) lights on during sex play	never/sometimes/often	never/sometimes/often
c) touching own genitals	never/sometimes/often	never/sometimes/often
d) touching partner's genitals	never/sometimes/often	never/sometimes/often
e) foreplay in bed (over 3 min)	never/sometimes/often	never/sometimes/often
f) new sexual positions	never/sometimes/often	never/sometimes/often
g) sexual discussion with partner	never/sometimes/often	never/sometimes/often
h) guilt around sex act	never/sometimes/often	never/sometimes/often
i) anxiety around sex act	never/sometimes/often	never/sometimes/often
j) shame about sex activity	never/sometimes/often	never/sometimes/often
k) enjoyment of sex play	never/sometimes/often	never/sometimes/often
l) enjoyment of sex act	never/sometimes/often	never/sometimes/often
m) frequency of masturbation	_____ times per month	_____ times per month
n) frequency of intercourse	_____ times per month	_____ times per month

5. About how frequently did they do the prescribed home sex play?
   per week: Week 1 _ Week 2 _ Week 3 _ Week 4 _ Week 5 _ Week 6 _ Week 7 _

6. Which factors do you think help the patient most? Score: 1 (least)...10 (most)

   a) partner's changed attitude: ___ Describe: _____

   b) therapist's intervention: ___ Describe: _____

   c) the physical _____
   d) the sexological _____
   e) the slides _____
   f) the home sex discussion _____
   g) the home sex play _____
   h) the program's pressure for action _____
   i) knowing other couples also had sex problems _____
   j) knowing other couples had succeeded _____
   k) other: ___ Describe: _____

partner. Two consultant gynecologists and two urologists are in attendance.

Home sensual loveplay (sensate focus) with no intercourse is suggested for the first 2 weeks. Videos on touching, masturbation, and the squeeze technique are shown in weeks 4 to 6. Nonverbal communication is enhanced by a special fourth session in which the team gives cues to the couple, guided by nurturant supervisors. This is followed by empty-chair Gestalt therapy in which partners are asked to address areas of conflict such as money, closeness, power, hurt, and loneliness. On the last night (week 7), we recapitulate, integrate, reinforce gains, and evaluate changes. We also offer a 1-hour follow-up in 8 weeks' time. Evaluation sheets completed at weeks 1 and 7 are shown in Figure 1. (This form may be used by anyone who wishes, with proper acknowledgment.)

The Clinic accepts only married couples. Singles are seen in all-male and all-female groups that meet 90 minutes weekly for six sessions with same-sex therapists (one of whom is a psychiatry resident) in a structured program that includes one pre-group evaluation and audiovisuals during the sessions. Modified individual sex therapy with psychiatry residents who have completed the Clinic elective is also available.

I regard symptom reversal to coital competence as a therapeutic success. Just as physicians were similar in symptomatology to other professionals, they were also just as likely as the comparison groups to get good results from sex therapy. The success rate among physicians was 80 percent for impotence, anorgasmia, and ISD (both sexes); and 90 percent for premature ejaculation. One of the two unconsummated physician marriages was consummated, as were 56 other unconsummated marriages in the Clinic's total population; 70 percent were consummated by week 7. Long-term outcome was unknown. Not one physician has ever returned the mailed annual follow-up sheet, although it is designed to ensure privacy. Perhaps it reminds them of the unwelcome patient role. Overall mail return for the follow-up is 10 to 15 percent.

Case Examples

While figures and statistics provide some global information about physician couples and sex therapy, some detailed case examples serve better to illuminate the typical problems encountered.

One irritable, angry female physician was a partner in an unconsummated marriage of 3 years' duration. Her healthy, wealthy but sexually inhibited and inexperienced lawyer husband of 37 was virginal and impotent. She had only recently had her first orgasm by masturbation. She saw artificial insemination as the solution. Both her parents and his wanted a grandchild. She had contempt for his feelings, refusing to allow him to visit the gynecologist with her to discuss insemination. He, on the other hand, refused to provide ejaculate at home; she preferred medical journals to his company at home, and was so uncomfortable with his friends that she would pretend to be called by the hospital to get away from them. She rejected foreplay: "Why can't we just have intercourse and be done?" His selective impotence was hardly surprising. She attended only two sessions at the Clinic; he completed the 7 weeks alone, learning much from audiovisuals, but the treatment was a failure. She illustrated the "Queen Bee" Syndrome: "Fertilize me, then drop dead." Eventually, the marriage was annulled.

Among other things, the foregoing example illustrates the point made in the earlier chapters by Gabbard and Menninger, that the physician's single-minded devotion to medicine may leave little time for sexual intimacy. Medical journals during meals and in the bedroom have been a focus of recurring conflict for the physician couples we have seen at the Clinic. One physician's wife described it as follows:

Wednesday night he'll say, "are you ready," place the journal open on the bedside table, finish intercourse in silence in 2 minutes, turn the light on again and complete his article, not caring at all about me. I haven't climaxed since our first child 17 years ago.

Another woman complained that her physician husband palpated her abdomen during loveplay as if he were doing a pelvic examination. Yet another comment, "It's like he even wears his stethoscope to bed! He never stops being a doctor!" One internist, who had no time for the formalities of courting, simply went to a computer video dating service after completing his residency and selected a wife, after determining that she was of acceptable religion and family.

A 35-year-old female physician said, "I really was never much for sex. I married my husband for companionship. As a linguistics professor he knew so much about history and literature. But now

we are fighting about sex all the time. Not that I refuse him
coitus, but he gets mad because I don't respond. Sometimes I
pretend. I have never told him that 2 years ago I learned how to
achieve an orgasm for the first time from one of those 'becoming
orgasmic' paperbacks that a patient must have left around. It
works for me, but I don't want to destroy his ego by telling him I
masturbate."

Many nonphysician wives use similar rationales for faking orgasm.
   Extramarital affairs are also a recurring theme in the complaints of physician couples.

A 45-year-old surgeon with selective impotence recounted the
following: "At the start of the marriage, I had premature
ejaculation, but after reading up on the 'squeeze technique,' we
applied it and it worked. That's not the problem now. Now she
says she's upset about my affair, drinking too much, and losing
my temper."

A striking finding is that alcohol abuse (past or current) is more
prevalent in male physicians who had affairs than in any of the
other professions (see Table 2). It is possible that physicians shed
their inhibitions only when they drink. An ophthalmology resident
contracted herpes and tried to convince his R.N. bride that it came
from a throat culture. He finally admitted to an affair; their marriage and sex life survived through therapy.
   Many physician couples are difficult patients. A nonsympto-
matic orthopedic resident dropped out of treatment after one visit,
despite his promise to his wife. She had primary orgasmic dysfunction and had earned the money to pay for the therapy as a
cocktail waitress. She came for one more session, then called to
say that her husband had accepted a position in Boston. She, with
two children, was to take care of packing and moving. Respect,
tolerance, and mutuality had no part in this physician's 5-year-
old marriage. His wife's need for sexual fulfillment was a nuisance
to him. Another female physician dropped out, but her husband
finished on his own, overcoming premature ejaculation. An attractive black woman lawyer insisted to her handsome black internist husband that she was among the 15 percent of women
identified by Masters and Johnson (1970) who had no interest in
ever having an orgasm; she did not change this attitude in the 7
weeks of treatment. Dozens of other vignettes could be cited that
indicate conflict about and resistance to treatment typical of many

medical couples. The course was generally smoother among my 77 solo physician patients, many of whom came after a divorce or the breakup of a love affair.

Physicians who accepted the patient role cooperated well, responded to treatment, and said they learned much about relating to their partner and about sexuality in general. A good sexual life can provide strong bonding and continuous reaffirmation of love. When there is a sexual problem, blame, helplessness, anxiety, resentments, and uncertainty will build up through the years.

Conclusion

My data indicate that the nature of sexual dysfunction in physician couples is not fundamentally different from that of other professionals. Fortunately, most of these problems are reversible. Which comes first: sexual symptoms or relationship problems? Often it is impossible to tell, so both must be treated simultaneously. Both may improve with effective sex therapy. In my work, medical colleagues receive the same treatment as all other couples. But many physician couples said that the 5 hours per week of the program, plus the hour of travel, was the longest time they had spent alone together in years! Their relationships improved as their sexual symptoms were cured. The physician's spouse (often for the first time) had a safe place to express feelings and to be heard. All of the patients had to make time to do their assigned sexual tasks at home. Time together and the sharing of arousal feelings are two special love gifts that modern couples can give each other. Quality time can truly compensate for scarce quantity.

It is rewarding to treat physician couples, for me and for the trainees. All of us learn valuable lessons, especially about marriages where sexual behavior indicates the level of disrepair. Intimacy is a lifelong desire and a challenge to the maturity of each partner. Each must recognize the other's dignity and rights so that normal differences and anger may be understood, expressed, and accepted. Honesty always brings the risk of being hurt; but emotional hurts, like physical ones, can be healed.

The Occupational Hazards of Having a Physician Father

Martin Leichtman, Ph.D.

Much research has been done on the psychological and marital problems of physicians and their spouses, but little attention has been paid to their children's problems. To be sure, studies note the disappointment and guilt physicians feel about not spending more time with their families (Bates and Moore 1975; Bergman 1980; Derdeyn 1978); and books by and about physicians' wives (Fine 1981; Smith 1980) invariably make some reference to child rearing. However, the problems are rarely explored in depth either in these books or in the psychiatric literature.

Here the "Physicians and Their Families" workshop (described in the Introduction) has provided a unique opportunity. Small group sessions invariably devoted considerable time and attention to the problems of child rearing. In addition, adolescents filled out questionnaires on the effects of medical careers on them, their siblings, and their parents. These issues were then explored in informal individual and group sessions, followed by a panel discussion in which some of the adolescents elaborated their ideas in response to their parents' questions.

Drawing on these sources as well as on clinical experience at The Menninger Clinic, I will examine in this chapter some of the problems encountered by children in the traditional American physician's family—one in which the husband pursues a full-time

The author thanks Dr. Maria Luisa Leichtman for her thoughtful critical review of this chapter.

medical career and the wife is chiefly a homemaker.* The first section will consider three aspects of the physician family and a distinct hazard inherent in each; the second section will explore ways in which these hazards affect children at different stages of their lives; and the conclusion will consider how these children and their families cope.

Medical Careers and Family Life

Physicians and Fatherhood:
The Physician as Part-Time Parent

Having spent much of his adolescence and young adulthood becoming a doctor, the physician makes that role the foundation of his self-definition, and meeting its demands determines most of his conduct. Although the physicians in our groups complain vigorously about work demands, community expectations, patient ingratitude, responsibilities, strain, and exhaustion, few feel that any other profession would be as satisfying.

Physicians find it hard to relinquish their professional roles in ordinary human relationships. At the workshop they joke about how doctors unsuccessfully try to treat their wives and children as they treat patients, staff, and colleagues. Children are affected by living with a parent whose profession exposes him to continual stress generated by constant exposure to the suffering of the sick and dying (McCue 1982). Children are also influenced by the physician personality patterns noted by Vaillant and others (Derdeyn 1978; Gabbard 1985; Vaillant et al. 1972), which are described in Chapter 3.

Participants in the workshop also emphasize something more concrete: the extraordinary capacity of medical practice to absorb

---

*The problems of children who have a physician for a mother will not be addressed here, partly because of the small size of our sample, and partly because the situation of these women is fundamentally different from that of male physicians. Men typically define themselves as physicians first and spouses and parents second. Women are less likely and less able to do that. Male physicians usually assume that their wives will handle most of the day-to-day parenting responsibilities. In contrast, women physicians typically have major responsibility for the home, and they often modify or curtail their careers to care for children (Heins et al. 1977a; Jussim and Muller 1975; Powers et al. 1969). Finally, whereas male physicians follow a common, almost stereotypical pattern of handling career–family conflicts, female patterns are far more diverse, and depend on the personalities and values of the marital partners. Hence, the hazards of having a physician for a mother are beyond the scope of this chapter.

time and attention. Elliot (1979) found that only 18 percent of her group of English hospital physicians spent 35 or more waking hours at home, as compared with 50 percent of dentists. These families know that a physician's socialization aims at inculcating a total devotion to medicine (Gerber 1983). They know that medical training blurs the distinction between work and overwork; that patients and colleagues later reinforce the will to put medicine first; and that the physician's own character structure and values reinforce these influences.

Thus the children of physicians have fathers who are often unavailable or tired, preoccupied, and inattentive. Even when engaged in family activities, they may be called away without notice. In addition to this work-related unavailability, there is the even more serious emotional aloofness and psychological unavailability that are aspects of the compulsive personality structure described in earlier chapters. In short, then, because medicine is often a career-and-a-half, doctors may be only half-time fathers.

Physicians' Wives: The Mother as a Parent-and-a-Half

Most children of physicians are raised by a mother whose identity centers on being a physician's wife (see Chapter 4). To be sure, at the workshop, wives often point out that they are more "liberated" than the last generation of doctors' wives. They are more ready to pursue careers and demand time from their husbands, and less inclined to subordinate themselves to their husbands and their husbands' careers. Yet by contemporary standards, most follow quite a traditional pattern while their children are growing up. Many have worked as nurses, teachers, and social workers and continue to pursue these professions part-time; but their careers are almost always subordinated to the primary role of being a doctor's wife and the mother of his children.

The early years of marriage often involve the establishment of a division of labor in which physicians' wives may assume more responsibility than wives of other professionals for maintaining the home, organizing the family's social life, and above all, rearing children. In fact, mothers of young children in our groups often feel like single parents. Their husbands are satisfied with being physicians, but they are ambivalent about being physicians' wives.

These women, trying to be a parent-and-a-half while struggling with feelings of loneliness and lack of support from their husbands, are under more strain and are more dissatisfied than many other mothers. Children may grow up seeking to alleviate chronic covert conflict and unhappiness.

Medicine and Career-Family Conflicts: Medicine as an In-Law

Although physicians like to describe medicine as a "jealous mistress," for their families it is more like a respected but domineering in-law. If medicine were simply a mistress, families would find it easier to express their anger, experience their unhappiness, and deal with their conflicts. Wives and children seldom tolerate a mistress, let alone defer to her for years. But physicians, their wives, and their children all accept the legitimacy of professional obligation and the sacrifice of family interests it often requires. As Fine (1981) noted, "A doctor's wife and children live with the reality that medicine is regarded with more deference and respect than is extended to any other family member" (p. 152). As a result, all members of the family are often deeply ambivalent about family conflicts.

These three sets of hazards are almost universal in physician's families. I will now consider them in relation to the stages of a child's development.

Growing up in Physicians' Families

Starting Out

Because doctors tend to marry late (Thomas 1976), the first years of their marriage usually coincide with medical school, internship, residency, and beginning practice. These are the years in which they begin to establish a professional identity. The demands of medicine on time and energy are at a peak; physicians' control over hours and energy is at a minimum; and doctors struggle to prove themselves by meeting the rigid expectations of training institutions. Thus all three hazards are greatest when doctors and their wives are deciding to have children and when the children are young and vulnerable.

Physicians' wives must also come to terms with a new identity in the early years. They enter marriage with their eyes open, having begun to learn about the demands of medicine and the unpredictability of their husbands' schedules during courtship. But there is a difference between knowing something and experiencing it. The first years of marriage require a difficult adjustment. The decision to have children then reinforces their definition of themselves as doctors' wives. Combining a full-time job and rearing young children is difficult under the best of circumstances; it is especially hard when husbands are not available either to help with day-to-day work or to provide encouragement and emotional support. Doctors' wives with children who try to pursue full-time work may doubt that they are doing either job right. Most women in our groups have decided to postpone, abandon, or at least sharply curtail their careers.

On the other hand, children open opportunities as well. In addition to the usual reasons for wanting children, physicians' wives may also hope that they will compensate for a lack of intimacy in the marriage. Children promise both companionship missing in their marriages and a career (motherhood) as meaningful and as important as their husbands'.

Problems begin during pregnancy. For wives, the accompanying physical and psychological changes may accentuate loneliness and vulnerability. Husbands may lose some of their wives' support, attention, and emotional refueling as the women turn attention inward toward themselves and the baby. The chief hazard of a medical career at this stage is that it may restrict mutual support and shared experience.

Infancy

Of the developmental tasks children negotiate in the first year (Bowlby 1969; Brazelton 1969; Emde and Robinson 1979; Mahler et al. 1975; Spitz 1965; Stern 1985), two are especially noteworthy: (1) maintaining homeostasis, regulating their internal systems as they exercise emerging perceptual, motor, and cognitive skills; and (2) achieving attachment to others and beginning to establish themselves as social beings. Both parents are important in helping infants to master these tasks. Typically it is mothers who play the vital role in the intimate systems that allow infants to regulate physiological patterns, modulate and shape affective responses, and develop perceptual-motor, cognitive, and early linguistic skills. Infants require reciprocity on a moment-by-moment basis as mothers help them interact with the world (Brazelton 1969; Brazelton and Als 1979; Stern 1977).

Fathers play a variety of roles in their children's lives even at this early stage (Lamb 1976, 1981), but two are of particular significance. First, they serve as "assistant mothers," helping to provide physical care and intense reciprocal interaction. Second, they provide emotional support and links with the outside world that are essential at a time when their homebound wives are likely to fear being swallowed up by the role of mother and by the children's needs.

During this period, both parents are likely to be exhilarated, deeply involved in their labors yet often overworked and exhausted as they deal with others (children and patients) whose dependence can offer intense narcissistic rewards, but can also be unreasonable and ungratefully demanding. Physicians find variety in their work and support from co-workers; mothers are more likely to feel trapped, with no external sources of support except their husbands, to whom they must look increasingly for praise, interest, excitement, and encouragement. Unfortunately, physicians may lack the time, energy, and commitment to provide this, and infants may be raised chiefly by tired, lonely, frustrated, and at times depressed mothers.

The Toddler Years

The second and third years are among the most exciting and most difficult. On the one hand, children display extraordinary growth in motor, cognitive, and social skills. They discover the world about them and become recognizable individuals. On the other hand, in terms of emotional drain and sheer labor, no other years are as hard for their parents. They roam the house freely, get into mischief, expose themselves to danger, and require constant attention. A powerful, preemptory striving to become an individual alternates with intense demandingness and clingingness. Family life seems to consist of constant skirmishes as children learn limits and master frustration, rage, and ambivalence toward those they love, even as they assert themselves. This intense interaction assists the child in the vital developmental task of establishing an identity (Brazelton 1974).

The impact on the family is apparent whenever parents meet. At the workshop, groups composed of couples with young children often feel set apart from other groups by the battle to domesticate their children. These parents are so absorbed in coping with the demands of their children that they often have little energy for anything else. Although they believe they ought to pursue a more exciting social life, they often prefer that the babysitter take the children out and let them have the house to themselves.

These are the years in which the fathers' limited availability may be hardest on both children and their mothers. During this phase, mothers have an even greater need for fathers as "assistants" and support systems than before. Because children are most deeply attached to their mothers, they typically reserve their angriest and most unreasonable behavior for them. Since fathers can provide the children with allies, alternate figures for identification, and a more positive, less emotionally charged parenting relationship (Brazelton 1974), they can exercise discipline without making children feel so angry and frustrated. Some physicians in our groups pride themselves on being able to deal easily with conflicts that stymie their wives. They mistakenly believe that their success is due to an ability to bring to child rearing the same firmness, patience, clarity of purpose, and rationality they employ in their medical practice. They are convinced that their wives could manage the children better if only they would adopt these approaches as well. But the real reason for their comparative success is that the children are eager for their attention and involved in less intense and hence less conflicted relationships with them. The longer fathers spend with toddlers, the harder they find it to maintain the consistency, patience, and rationality they value.

The chief hazard to physicians' children at this age is that their fathers may have little time and energy for them. As a result, three patterns of difficulties in mother–child relationships often emerge.

The first and perhaps most common is a rather dependent, depressed mother and a child who shows "anxious attachment" (Bowlby 1973), or has problems with "separation" (Mahler et al. 1975). Feeling that her husband does not offer enough help, such a mother is deeply troubled by the fearfulness, inhibitions, nightmares, sleep problems, tantrums, and other expressions of conflict characteristic of children at this age. She often hopes that the child's problems will draw her husband's attention away from medicine, even if it means an argument.

In one of the workshops, for example, attention focused on this pattern.

> Mrs. R., a woman in her late 20s, felt inadequate as a mother because of the fearfulness, sleep disturbances, crying, and clinging of her daughter, a shy, inhibited 2-year-old. Acutely

sensitive to her daughter's own helpless dependency and
difficulty in separating, Mrs. R. strongly identified with the child.
She felt desperately in need of help her husband could not or
would not give. Dr. R. felt overworked, depressed, and trapped
by the demands of his practice. He felt guilty not only about
neglecting family, but also about not doing enough for his
parents. Both he and his wife were concerned that he saw his
family merely as one more drain on his already overtaxed
resources.

Other couples at the workshop were especially sensitive to such
difficulties, because they are exaggerated forms of problems familiar to most physician families.

A second problematic pattern is one in which the wife is openly
angry and frustrated with her husband and child. In these cases,
the main conflicts involve the child's aggressiveness, opposition-
alism, and readiness to act up. The child's symptoms may be a
vehicle for the expression of the mother's anger; the mother may
treat the child as the father's surrogate; or the child may be used
as a "hostage" to coerce the father into greater family involvement. Often the parents use erratic forms of discipline, intensi-
fying the child's own problems with aggression and self-control.

A third pattern, in which the child lives out the frustrated
aspirations of the mother, may provoke a new generation to re-
produce the problems of the old. In these cases, the mother is
closely attuned to the needs of her child; eager to foster talents,
competence, and sensitivity; and ready to facilitate the process of
individuation. With a first child in particular, the mother must
encourage independence because younger children are on the way.
However, the process of individuation is subtly distorted. When
a woman has sacrificed her own career and goals, the child is
"special," becoming the carrier of her own aspirations and the
proof of her creativity as a parent. A child who seems mature and
sensitive from an early age can also become a source of comfort
and companionship to the mother, filling a vacuum left by her
husband. Such "specialness" has a price. True autonomy, the freedom to pursue one's own life, is reduced. Meanwhile the child is
pressured to ignore and deny regressive or dependent wishes while
constantly striving to succeed. The child's character structure may
then begin to resemble the father's. Not surprisingly, many doctors in our group were themselves children of doctors.

The Preschool Years

In this period children develop a greater capacity for representational thought, a broadened time sense, a deepening experience of themselves and their worlds, and an increasingly rich play and fantasy life (Heinicke 1979). They continue to establish themselves as autonomous beings and to consolidate character traits and defensive patterns. Clearly defined gender identities emerge; they experiment with social roles in play and fantasy; they internalize parental values; and they move beyond dyadic relationships with parents to increasingly complex, triangular ones (Silverman et al. 1975; Solnit 1979).

Now they experience their fathers and their fathers' profession differently. Like police officers and firefighters, and unlike lawyers, accountants, and psychologists, doctors have a profession that children can understand. They see the importance of their fathers' work and become ready to credit them with a healing power that amplifies the already strong inclination of children of this age to idealize their fathers. At the same time, they now recognize more clearly the disappointments they suffer from their fathers' absence, unpredictability, and emotional distance. They also understand better the conflicts between their parents, and this shapes their fantasies about themselves and their roles in the family system.

One problem at this age is the consolidation of gender identity. While a core gender identity, a sense of whether one is a boy or a girl, probably develops even earlier (Money and Ehrhardt 1972; Stoller 1975), during these years the sense of *what kind* of a boy or girl one is becomes established (Jacobson 1964). For boys in particular, positive father–child relationships facilitate the emergence of a healthy gender identity and successful heterosexual relationships later in life; inadequate father–child relationships and the absence of fathers from the home interfere with this process (Biller 1981a, 1981b). Physicians' families are often sensitive to this problem (Elliot 1979). At the workshop, parents of preschool children frequently stress that "boys need a father" and express concerns about shyness, inhibition, and "effeminacy." In other cases, a boy's sense of maleness is stimulated by being treated as "the man of the family" in the father's absence. Such a role is uncertain because it must be supported by yet more powerful females. Where the marriages are strong, physicians' wives make special efforts to maintain contact between sons and fathers. For example, they let children stay up when fathers work late and give up family time to assure that fathers and sons have time together.

Preschoolers are eager to get their fathers' attention, show off projects, and gain recognition. Therefore, fathers can influence their development profoundly. Because of the importance they attribute to their fathers and their fathers' work, physicians' children are especially open to such influences. Yet children have a harder time translating ambitions into reality when fathers are absent or too tired and preoccupied to be adequate models, teachers, and audiences. Furthermore, the standards children set for themselves now in the hope of winning parental love and recognition are prototypes of the standards they will set for themselves as adults. They tend to develop ego ideals heavily influenced by their parents' emphasis on work, achievement, and self-sacrifice. Yet because their fathers are less available, these ego ideals will be less realistic and attainable than those of other children. When nothing they do gives them sufficient attention from their fathers, talented youngsters may doubt their worth even as they drive themselves to achieve in order to demonstrate that they are special. For some youngsters, the unattainable ego ideal fuels the pursuit of perfection described in Chapter 3 and can contribute to overt depression later in life.

Finally, the limited availability of physicians to their families may have a profound effect on the oedipal conflicts and "triangular" relationships that influence children's personalities during these years. The role of "man of the house" may leave boys overstimulated, guilty, and struggling with anxieties about filling shoes too big for them. Girls may idealize physician fathers as romantic figures with whom they have brief periods of intimacy alternating with longer periods of distance and seeming indifference. Psychoanalysts have long believed that the handling of such conflicts is decisive in personality formation.

Meanwhile the family structure and the role of children within it are crystallizing. In medical families, these are often years of marital disillusionment. Physicians have outside sources of satisfaction; their wives often do not. As a result, mothers and children may band together to exclude fathers from family life; or children, sensitive to their parents' unhappiness, may be placed in or adopt roles designed to meet their parents' needs and balance the family system. Hence, they participate in the "triangles" discussed in Chapter 11.

Middle Childhood

Compared with earlier and later stages, the elementary school years are relatively easy. Because of their growing maturity, hormonal changes, cognitive development, and shifts of interests beyond the home, latency-age children become more reasonable and less demanding (Powell 1979). Everyday pressures diminish because children are in school much of the time and the family is less the center of their existence. Parents in our groups note these changes with some ambivalence, joking about their demotion to taxi driver, short-order cook, or valet, but also recognizing that their lives have become easier. In addition, problems related to achievement and movement into a broader social world may be affected by having a physician for a father.

Learning, achieving, and developing talents are now increasingly important to children. The goals children set for themselves play a central role. Fathers continue to serve as models, teachers, and audiences. When asked about the disadvantages of having a doctor for a father, teenagers often recalled "broken promises" and disappointments from this period of life—school activities, Little League games, plays, and recitals their fathers were too busy to attend. Mothers described (somewhat resentfully) having to "fill in" for fathers at such activities.

In some cases, children keep searching for what is missing within the family and lack the confidence to move beyond these relationships into a world of peers and other adults.

For example, one 10-year-old at the workshop was a lonely, inhibited boy who depended heavily on his family and had great difficulty making friends. Asked about the advantages of having a physician for a father, he said that you could always count on good care when you were sick. He had complained for years about symptoms with no clear physical basis; he apparently believed that only by becoming a patient could he get attention from his father, not unlike the behavior of the wives of some physicians noted in Chapter 4.

On the other hand, adolescents often suggest an advantage in their fathers' absence: they learn greater self-reliance and independence. Some say they model themselves on their fathers in this respect. There is an undercurrent of regret in these remarks, as if they had hoped for more but had learned they had to "grow up." Many feel they have to depend on themselves alone; some are able to turn to teachers, coaches, relatives, siblings, and friends for attention and recognition. In their absence, physicians do pay a price here, for these years are among the best that parents have to enjoy with their children.

Adolescence

Adolescence is, above all, a period of transition. At its outset, children live within and define themselves in relation to their families; at its conclusion, they are expected to move out, ready to manage their own lives and define themselves as quasi-independent persons in relation to society (Petersen and Offer 1979). While still dependent on their parents for support and direction, adolescents often need to repudiate much of what their parents have to offer and to rely instead on peers, teachers, mentors, and, in the end, themselves. They must discover their talents, learn to accept their limitations, and find ways to regulate self-esteem (Malmquist 1979). In forging their identities, they must try to resolve conflicts rooted in their childhood, accept or reject parental identifications, and choose which of their parents' values they will live by (Erikson 1968).

Adolescents' independence also alters the identities of their parents. Adolescents need to know not only whether they can manage without their parents, but also whether their parents can manage without using them as a peacekeeping buffer, a lightning rod for conflict, a source of comfort, and so forth. They must face doubt and guilt about leaving their mothers with empty lives. Parents now realize that they are becoming "dispensable." If they have organized their identities around parenting, they must learn to think differently about themselves and find other ways to give meaning to their lives.

Adolescent children of physicians face further problems that reflect the impact of their father's profession. They must come to terms with both its positive and its negative effects. They must discover whether they are strong enough and their relationship good enough for them to accept what their fathers have provided and forgive them for what was not. They must find out to what extent they can share or must repudiate their fathers' dedication to hard work, sense of duty, and high standards. If they do use these identifications, they must see how much they do so in rigid defensive ways to counter unmet dependency needs and deny frustration and disappointment. They must discover whether these standards are realistic for them or will leave them with a sense of inadequacy.

Adolescents must also come to terms with the manner in which their fathers' careers have affected their mothers; they must make use of what their mothers have given them and accept the inevitable failures. Adolescent identities will often be shaped by a wish to ease their mothers' burdens, often by "parenting" themselves and their siblings.

Finally, adolescents must master their own ambivalence about the medical ethic of self-sacrifice, duty, and denial of personal concerns and its cost to family and children. Those who have good relationships with their fathers and strong families may embrace such values, accepting the costs. Others embrace this ethic only in a deeply ambivalent manner. Still others may have such a troubled relationship with their families that they repudiate and denigrate both medical and family values.

Three types of adolescents with varying degrees of problems can be identified. First, most adolescents who accompany their parents to the workshop appear to have negotiated the hazards well. Displaying the pattern of "continuous growth" that Offer and Offer (1975) described as the most common route through normal adolescence, they work hard to present themselves as "typical American teenagers." They are doing reasonably well in school and have friends. Despite minor battles with their parents, they retain a strong family loyalty. Many described their homes in ways reminiscent of old-fashioned television shows like "Father Knows Best." They acknowledged problems but also sought to deny or, at least, minimize them before an audience of parents. The denial was so great that the panel of adolescents was eventually dropped from the workshop program because so many punches were being pulled.

These are adolescents who try to be the children their parents wish them to be, albeit with some ambivalence. For some, this means overcompliance, denial of their own needs, and a readiness to pursue ideals beyond their reach. Others reach such accommodations comfortably. If their lives seem too conformist for some tastes, those who live and work closely with adolescents know that things could be much worse.

A second type of adolescent is crippled by efforts to cope with family problems.

An example is Kurt, a serious, rather depressed 16-year-old who accompanied his parents to one of the workshops. Although bright and hungry for relationships with peers, Kurt was a chronic underachiever in school, inhibited and preoccupied with the family. In discussions with the other teenagers, he showed exquisite sensitivity to the problems posed by his father and his father's work. He spoke movingly of his disappointments; the difficulty of living up to his father's expectations; his efforts to help his unhappy, overworked mother; and the effect of family tensions on his sibling.

His father stood out in a group of 25 physicians because he flaunted his overriding commitment to medical values above all else. He actually embarrassed the others, who saw him as a caricature of the ideal physician. Kurt's mother was deeply unhappy, masochistically assuming the burden imposed by her husband's career. Physicians and wives in this group spent much of the workshop trying to help the family, but Kurt's father seemed indifferent to what they said.

The leaders of the group hoped that during the adolescent panel Kurt's father might finally listen. It was not to be. When Kurt spoke, he kept his eyes on his father and endorsed fully his father's values and style of life, while the father beamed with pleasure. Undoubtedly, Kurt feared his father's displeasure and desperately wanted his approval. But he probably also felt protective, sensing that the man's rigidity was accompanied by fragility and extreme vulnerability. After the panel, Kurt seemed deeply depressed. He shared privately some of his feelings and was amenable to suggestions of counseling or psychotherapy.

Kurt's case shows why some physicians' children may be unable to grow up and live their own lives. Instead, they are depressed and inhibited underachievers because they have not received enough attention to their developmental needs. They identify with standards with which they cannot live. They are trapped in a constricting role as they try to mediate conflicts between their parents and alleviate family unhappiness at the cost of their own growth.

A third pattern involves more seriously disturbed behavior with an outright repudiation of both medical and family values.

This pattern is illustrated by Bruce, a 15-year-old who was referred for a comprehensive psychiatric evaluation because of chronic delinquency and drug use. Bruce did not come from the kind of family that attended workshops on the problem of balancing commitments to medicine and family. To the contrary, his father, a busy orthopedic surgeon, would not even come for Bruce's evaluation until a court gave him a choice between doing so or seeing his son placed in a detention home because of stealing and drug dealing. The father made it clear that he had little time for his family and that he expected his wife to handle child rearing. Bruce's mother was angry about these expectations, bitterly unhappy with her marriage, and resentful toward her son who had seemed to her an aggressive, demanding child since birth. She stayed in the marriage only because of the family's wealth and position in the community.

In the course of the evaluation, it became clear that Bruce's antisocial attitudes were, in part, a commentary on his parents' lives. The family continually stressed that his father's work made possible the material benefits he enjoyed. Angry about his father's neglect, he assumed that money and possessions were his due; he took them without gratitude, squandered them, and demanded more. When younger, he had sometimes been sensitive to his mother's unhappiness. In adolescence he felt only contempt for what he saw to be her weakness and for her concern about community status, which he rejected by engaging in publicly antisocial activities. Bruce dismissed his father's claims about the value of his work as blatant hypocrisy and insisted that he cared only for money, power, and attention. He said that their family life was no more than a front.

Bruce's father viewed treatment chiefly as a medical problem to be turned over to others while he returned to his practice. Bruce's mother also wanted to leave her son to have whatever was wrong with him "fixed." Bruce had no intention of being "cured" under such circumstances. The deeply rooted antisocial tendencies in this boy were continually accentuated by his anger at and disappointment with his parents and their lives.

This is not to attribute such pathology to the impact of medical careers alone. Obviously, the problems of physicians' children are heavily influenced by constitution, life history, parents' characters, and other factors. Kurt and Bruce might have had many of the same problems if their fathers had been accountants, plumbers, or used car salesmen. What I am suggesting is that the specific hazards of having a physician for a parent interact with these other factors, and play a significant role in how adolescents come to terms with their past and how they forge their futures.

Conclusion

In this chapter, I have argued that the chief "occupational hazards" of having a physician for a father arise from the fact that the extraordinary amount of time, energy, and attention that the physician devotes to his career often comes at the cost of lack of time and energy to invest in family life, a problem often compounded by the physician's compulsive personality. As a result, physicians' children may be angry, depressed, and frustrated. Moreover, because their own values so strongly support the demands of medical practice, all members and especially the children of physicians' families may be deeply conflicted.

While families at the workshop articulate the problems these hazards pose for children at each stage of their development, they also indicate strengths that enable physicians and their families to compensate for the costs of medical careers and to cope with the problems confronting them. In the relatively traditional families at the workshop, a number of factors appear to contribute to healthy development in children. First and most important is the psychological strength of the mother and her satisfaction with the roles of physician's wife and parent-and-a-half. The healthier families often center on mothers who do not allow legitimate dissatisfaction with their burdens to spill over into their relationships with their children. In our groups, the children doing best have active, energetic mothers who thrive on having children; find time for jobs, hobbies, social activities, and community involvement; and are able to support their husbands as well. Such mothers facilitate fathers' contacts with their children and are sensitive to ways in which they can substitute for their husbands when work interferes with their participation in the children's lives.

Secondly and almost as important is the father's love for and investment in his wife and his children. "Quality time" is not a substitute for quantity, but it is important. Fathers who are responsive to their family's needs, set aside time for them, and convey their affection and interest make significant contributions even in limited interactions. By providing their wives and children with tangible signs of care, recognition for their talents, and appreciation for their struggles, they become a positive presence in the home even when they are at work, and they help their families accept the sacrifices needed for their medical careers.

Third, the health of the marriage affects the children's lives. To the extent that the marital relationship is a comfortable and satisfying one, parents have less need to draw their children into parental roles that interfere with healthy development.

Finally, inborn strengths and character of children are critical: their talents; their capacity to tolerate frustration and disappointment; the use they are able to make of what their parents offer; and their ability to get from siblings, extended family, peers, and neighbors what their fathers do not provide. As children grow older, their capacity to recognize the value of their fathers' work helps them to accept their own sacrifices. Adolescents on panels at the workshop were so eager to convey this message that the panels were almost too comfortable an experience for their parents.

There are no easy prescriptions for the quality of life in medical families. In one sense, the problems are not soluble. The demands of family and career cannot be entirely reconciled. What constitutes a livable solution for one family may not be so for others. Programs like the "Physicians and Their Families" workshop do not offer particular solutions, but they do provide physicians and their wives with time together and an opportunity to rethink and renegotiate basic issues of family life.

The Medical Marriage at Midlife

Glen O. Gabbard, M.D.
Roy W. Menninger, M.D.

> Beware of what you dream to be in your youth for you will
> become that thing in your middle-age.
> > —Johann Wolfgang von Goethe

In *The Hospital*, a 1971 film directed by Arthur Hiller, George C. Scott plays Dr. Herb Bock, an academic physician in the throes of midlife crisis. Early in the screenplay (for which Paddy Chayefsky won an Academy Award), Dr. Bock drops in on a psychiatrist colleague (David Hooks). Opening with an acknowledgment that he is "not good at confessional," Bock describes his recent struggles with depression. He goes on to recount a childhood and adolescence marked by intellectual brilliance and social ineptitude. He characterizes his marriage as "sadomasochistic dependency" and remarks that he is not sure if he is impotent since he hasn't tried to make love in years. He is filled with self-recrimination for neglecting his children, who have drifted into revolutionary politics and drug pushing. He ruminates about the proper dose of potassium that would result in death but still give him time to dispose of the syringe so as to avoid conjecture about suicide. His self-disclosure to his psychiatric colleague embarrasses him, and he rushes out in the middle of it, hurrying back to work.

Most of the classic features of midlife crisis are captured in this vivid dialogue. This brilliant, overachieving physician comes to the midpoint of his life with his youthful dreams of glory crashing down around his head. His marriage is in a shambles. His children disappoint him. Profound depression is leading him to thoughts of suicide. He is filled with guilt about his failure to exercise parental responsibility. It has been a long time since he has attempted to make love with his wife. While the adjustments of middle age cause a normal period of regression and depression in most adults, the physician may be particularly vulnerable. As Waring (1974) noted: "Obsessionality, lack of pleasure-seeking, and feelings of indispensability while being useful as a student and fitting 'the good doctor' role may predispose to affective disorder in middle life" (p. 523). This is also the rockiest period for the medical marriage. Rose and Rosow (1972) found that the largest percentage (20.6 percent) of physician couples were divorced between the ages of 35 and 44, at the height of the physician's career.

Issues of Midlife

The midlife crisis is so thoroughly popularized in our culture of narcissism that it has become something of a cliché. Its psychological and physiological features in males were summed up by Brim (1976):

> The hormone production levels are dropping, the head is balding, the sexual vigor is diminishing, the stress is unending, the children are leaving, the parents are dying, the job horizons are narrowing, the friends are having their first heart attacks, the past floats by in a fog of hopes not realized, opportunities not grasped, women not bedded, potentials not fulfilled, and the future is a confrontation with one's own mortality. (p. 3)

The midlife period, between 35 and 55 years of age, brings with it the awareness that there is more life already lived than yet to be lived. Psychoanalytic writers on this subject are indebted to Erik Erikson (1963), who first defined the developmental task of midlife as a dialectic between stagnation and generativity. Colarusso and Nemiroff (1979), in their systematic psychoanalytic observations on adult development, emphasized the increasing awareness of the finiteness of time and of one's own mortality. They elaborated on the severe narcissistic injury inherent in aging—with its wrinkles, hair loss, decreased sexual drive, declining physical stamina—and the sobering realization that one's goals and dreams will only be partially achieved. In his classic 1965 paper, Elliot Jaques linked the task of midlife to the working through of the depressive position: the middle-aged man must come to terms with his own death and his potential for destructiveness toward those he loves.

As we emphasized in Chapter 3, physicians often engage in a perpetual quest for a transcendent state of perfection where aggression, greed, selfishness, and hatred are vanquished. Midlife confronts physicians with the impossibility of that goal. They have unsuccessfully tried to please everyone with self-sacrifice and now ask, "Where is the reward?" After postponing gratification since childhood, they discover that no reward can measure up to their expectations. Material rewards bring temporary gratification, but start to ring hollow in midlife. The rewards of patient gratitude and appreciation come to be seen as inadequate as well. Physicians often find that their needs and patients' needs are different. Physicians want to cure, but patients may wish to hang on to their symptoms to maintain dependency on the physician. As Derdeyn (1978) commented, midlife physicians are likely to feel dissatisfied and angry with the practice of medicine, as though they have been jilted by the "mistress" who has been the focus of every waking minute.

All these problems may come to a head in a crisis, such as a malpractice suit. Malpractice suits are devastating partly because of their unconscious meaning. It is as though the doctor's repressed aggressive wishes have suddenly been laid bare for all to see. The physician thinks the well-constructed defense of caring for others has been exposed as a sham. The physician fears being regarded as sadistic and neglectful. As Jaques (1965) pointed out, coming to terms with the destructiveness in all close human relationships is a key developmental task in midlife.

As the physician sinks progressively into the quagmire of midlife despair, existential issues become a prominent consideration. Like the ditchdigger, the banker, the garbage collector, and the millionaire, the physician comes to recognize the inevitability of death. Before, that realization could be fended off by youthful manic defenses. Now it begins to haunt the physician with each unrelenting tick of the clock, underscored by the deaths of friends and parents. Fundamental questions of meaning arise that the physician had hoped the very nature of medical practice would resolve. The physician asks, "Why am I here? What is my ultimate purpose? How can I find meaning or redemption in my life? How do I confront death with courage?" If neither work nor accumulation of wealth delivers meaning to one's life, what does?

Physicians respond in a variety of ways. A period of regressive behavior and depression, expectable in almost everyone, may intensify and become pathological. Some pathological responses include excessive and inappropriate physical activity, denial of age-appropriate needs and interests, renewed interest in the youth culture (including sex with much younger partners), job changes in midcareer, divorce, love affairs, flight into overwork, retreat into dogma, and rigidity. The ubiquitous depression may lead to suicide in the most severe cases. Mourning is the best resolution of midlife crisis (Jaques 1965). In seeking help, many physicians ask, "What can I *do*?" But the answer lies in reflection rather than action. In the first half of life, activity is a successful defense, but it tends to lose its effectiveness in middle age. If one allows time to reassess one's values and goals, and to grieve over the losses associated with aging, the midlife passage can strengthen the ego and deepen the character. However, physicians (and others as well) often prefer replacement to mourning. Instead of going through the painful grief process, they may think, "If only I had a different spouse, if only I were in a different specialty, if only I worked harder," etc.

Impulsive changes may be the most destructive course of all, as the case of Dr. H. shows.

> Dr. H. was a 44-year-old obstetrician who requested psychotherapy when his professional and personal life became unbearable. His practice had been miserable for 14 years, and his marriage had been unhappy for the full 16 years. He was a compulsive workaholic who had dutifully put up with all this as an unavoidable obligation. He grew up burdened with high expectations. He painfully remembered an incident in the sixth grade when his father was helping him with homework. The young boy was unable to grasp a concept in his science lesson, and his father became so frustrated that he threw the book at him yelling, "You'll never amount to anything!" As long as he could remember, Dr. H. had always felt that he was not fulfilling the expectations of his parents.
>
> Dr. H. was also consumed with guilt about his anger with his parents. When he went off to college, his mother started to nag him about how much he was changing. At the end of his freshman year, his mother became seriously ill. After returning to

see her in her hospital bed, he decided to transfer to a local college near home and to change his major to premed. In psychotherapy, he came to realize that he had felt responsible for his mother's illness and had gone home to make reparation. Becoming a physician while his mother was gravely ill was a way of unconsciously repairing the damage.

In the years before his midlife crisis, Dr. H. had been in charge of an obstetrics service in a large community hospital. He tried to create a situation in which he could avoid all feelings of guilt by performing flawlessly. He was extremely concerned about the malpractice crisis and had worked long hours implementing a fail-safe system in which mistakes would be impossible. He felt responsible for his colleagues' work as well as his own and tried to cover for their mistakes, making himself miserable in the process.

He was no better able to control guilt in his personal life. At the age of 34, he had had a brief affair with a nurse. He felt extraordinary guilt about this lapse, even though his marriage was barren and unhappy, and he speculated in psychotherapy that his depression might be self-punishment for that affair. The guilt had become so intense that a month before seeking psychotherapy, he impulsively confessed the affair to his wife, knowing that she would probably divorce him. He thought that the confession was a further self-punishment.

The preference for punishment from an external source, such as one's wife, to punishment by one's own harsh superego is a common dynamic in the psychology of the physician. Dr. H. sought help only when both his personal and professional lives were in serious jeopardy. He had been counterdependent in his choice of medicine as a career and belatedly realized in midlife that his dependency needs were not being met. He found himself questioning all the choices he had ever made and wondering whether a new direction in life was the answer. He no longer felt sure of anything he believed in. Like the George C. Scott character in *The Hospital*, even though he was preoccupied with suicide, he found it very difficult to ask for help. Bittker (1976) observed that physicians feel guilty about needing help because they have always maintained self-esteem through self-denial. Some physicians will commit suicide rather than request a psychiatric consultation. Sargent (1985) noted that two-thirds of physicians successfully commit suicide on their first attempt, a far higher rate of success than is found in any other comparable group.

The Marital Relationship at Midlife

Marriages too evolve through a series of stages. Berman and Lief (1975) described six stages, from young adulthood into middle adulthood. The task in Stage 1 is to break from families of origin and shift the primary commitment to the spouse. In Stage 2 there is uncertainty about the choice of one's spouse and stress caused by parenthood. During Stage 3 spouses may become restless as their rates of growth diverge, particularly if one spouse still has conflicting ties to the family of origin. In Stage 4 the primary task is productivity, in terms of both children and work. Husband and wife may have differing ways of achieving and viewing productivity. The marital task of the midlife transition, coinciding with Stage 5, is to sum up the past successes and failures and to evaluate goals. Now there are often differing perceptions of success and a conflict between individual achievements and commitment to the marriage. In Stage 6 the main task is stabilizing the marriage and healing wounds to make it durable. Taylor et al. (1983) proposed a similar scheme, in which they identified a career plateau after a period of maximum career demands has established the physician in practice. Physicians are sobered by the recognition that they have reached a peak professionally and that there is nowhere else to go.

In midlife the consequences of postponement in both spouses are finally felt. After repeated confrontations over intimacy, child rearing, responsibility around the house, in-laws, sexual relations, and other issues, the marital partners may have taken more and more divergent paths. It becomes increasingly difficult to preserve the fantasy that things will be better tomorrow. Many couples find themselves in two different worlds. They rarely have a meaningful exchange, may have stopped making love, and stay in the marriage mostly out of inertia. One middle-aged general practitioner said:

> We have had to stay together because our marriage is oriented around our children. We have one girl and three boys, and they mean a lot to us since we lost two of our first three children. My practice is old and boring, and it's way off in volume. Since I now have two partners, the practice is much easier than it used to be. My wife talks a lot while I don't talk enough. I find it difficult at times to express true thoughts and deep feelings. Consequently, there is a certain intimacy that's lacking which I could have with my wife. However, I know it's my fault.

His wife said:

> I have tried for so many years to be the perfect wife, mother,
> daughter, and daughter-in-law, etc. I have played "peace at any
> price" to the point of counting the years until our youngest was
> out of high school and we could go our separate ways. I guess I
> love him but now find myself with a separate successful career
> and two on the back burner, other sources of income besides my
> 40-hour-a-week job, a list of possible husbands (should anything
> happen to this one), and other friends. We have very few mutual
> friends, we never go out, and we never do things as a couple. We
> eat dinner around the same table, sometimes we cook together,
> and we occasionally have good sex. I am learning to be more
> vocal and to express my feelings, but this really upsets him. I
> want to be a married woman and would prefer to remain
> married to the man I have invested 28 years of my life in. When
> he laughs, it is like a miracle. My spouse seems to carry around
> this big cloud and wallow in misery. We do well in a crisis. I stop
> everything and totally attend to him. Then the crisis is over and I
> feel left at the station. I used to plan weekends alone, but I've
> quit. Now I plan to be with a friend, when I can feel intimacy
> and good about myself. I fantasize a lot and develop other
> relationships and make excuses to remain in this relationship. I
> still have hope and a strong sense of commitment. Someday he'll
> look at me and ask, "Where's my young wife?" I'll respond, "She
> got old waiting for you."

The Traditional Marriage

The divergent paths of the husband and wife in the traditional
marriage follow largely unconscious scripts that become apparent
in midlife. Robert May (1980) extensively studied gender patterns
in fantasy formation. A typical male fantasy is meteoric rise to
success leading to pride and self-importance, followed by a disastrous fall. The characteristic female fantasy is one of long-suffering loss and sorrow leading to a happy ending with a joyous
return to fullness and growth. Stories told by men on the Thematic
Apperception Test move from enhancement to deprivation; stories
told by women tend to move from deprivation to enhancement.
This pattern develops in middle childhood and is firmly established by late adolescence. These fantasy patterns may turn into
life scripts that become self-fulfilling prophecies in midlife.

The male physician has often been diligently establishing his
identity as an autonomous professional while neglecting intimate
relationships. The traditional wife has devoted herself to caring

for her husband and children, and often parents or parents-in-law as well. By their middle years both partners often feel that they have made extensive sacrifices and compromises for the sake of the marriage and family. Each feels unappreciated. Many years may have passed without much expression of affection or gratitude. The traditional wife may begin to feel depressed about having no identity except mother and wife. In addition to a neglectful husband, she may have rebellious adolescent children seeking to break the very ties she has spent her life developing. Zemon-Gass and Nichols (1975) found that the self-images of these women are vulnerable to the passage of time. Many women give up on their husbands in midlife, realizing that pursuit of intimacy with them is futile, and turn to school or work to forge a new identity. Meanwhile, the physician husband may belatedly return to his wife for the emotional intimacy that he missed, but she is now not as available to her husband as he would like her to be. He sinks into midlife despair; she becomes euphoric as she immerses herself in the new beginning. This midlife crossover pattern described by Bev Menninger in Chapter 5 is an extremely common form of marital disturbance in midlife.

The male physician has usually used activity as one of his main defensive strategies. As Jaques (1965) noted, this begins to falter in midlife, and anxiety starts to break through. David Gutmann (1964) studied the role of activity through the Thematic Apperception Test. According to Gutmann, as men age they tend to shift from "active mastery," a stage of self-initiated action, to "passive mastery," which means a stance of "resigned accommodation." The midlife male becomes more oriented toward internal change. Gutmann confirms the impression both of Jaques and of May (1980) that the male fantasy may moderate with age. In May's terms, the fantasy of prideful achievement is tempered with caring. Gutmann noted that this shift allows males to give and receive affection more easily.

Gutmann's (1964) work also provides some corroborating evidence for the crossover pattern. Aging in women seems to liberate dormant wishes for self-assertion and dominance. In other words, men and women move toward each other psychologically. The man starts to integrate his long-suppressed maternal or feminine side while the woman becomes more comfortable with the aggressive side of her nature.

If the traditional wife does not find a new identity, she may feel that life is passing her by. One physician's wife reported:

My husband is currently going through a midlife crisis, I think. He will turn 40 in June and is contemplating a career change. I have been in a life crisis for the past 2 years. In my heart and mind, I know my place is in the home with my four children. However, I feel unfulfilled and frustrated. I am floundering! I believe changes are very necessary, but I'm not sure if drastic ones would make an adequate difference. My favorite hobby is needlework. I think I'd like to earn money from this interest. There is no need for another needlework shop in my community, and I don't know if I'd want to run a shop anyway. I'd like some direction in my life other than mom and housewife, too. I'd like my own identity and my own money. I've never felt that my husband's salary is "our money" even though he's generally quite generous. As I say this, I feel stupid. I have so much to feel thankful for, yet I want more.

When the children leave home, the traditional wife may feel that she is floundering even more. Moreover, when husband and wife have used the children as a barrier to intimacy, they may be terrified at the prospect of facing each other alone every night. Some physicians, still fearing such emotional closeness, may decide that starting a new career is the answer. As one midlife physician said:

Recently I've been through a period of depression about turning 40. I'm dissatisfied with my practice. I took up some hobbies only to discover that I really like to work and prefer productive activity to idle conversation, playing games with children, etc. My wife accuses me of being greedy or going through a stage, but I don't think that is the case. My patient loads have dropped, my income has dropped, and my enthusiasm for my practice has fallen off. I have more time off, but I don't necessarily spend the time with my wife or children. I miss the challenge to my life. I wonder if I'm still capable of conquering tasks. Therefore, I'm in the process of applying for a new residency, and my wife feels betrayed, that is, her security and the children's future are undermined. I certainly don't want to lose any of them, but I feel that this change is necessary for me; and with their support we can all grow from the experience. Without their support it could mean problems for all of our futures, and I do not wish that to happen. I'm afraid to maintain the status quo for me, because I feel like I'm dying inside; but I don't want to make a change just for the sake of changing. I realize this isn't good timing with the ages of my children.

This physician's wife was upset by this:

> I had never seriously considered the possibility of separation in
> our marriage until the last several days. My husband, on his own
> and without consulting me, started a process of applying for a
> residency (after 16 years of practice). I became aware of it when
> one of the people he asked for a reference called our home with a
> question. My husband said he wanted to avoid the conflict and
> disagreement in discussing his actions with me until after he
> found out if any programs might be interested in him. This
> deeply hurt me, and my response was anger. He was correct in
> assuming that I would be against the move. It would involve
> changing schools for two of our three children when they are
> approaching graduation from high school. It would involve
> moving the whole family twice in 3 years, and would place us in
> a tenuous financial position of having several children in college
> while starting a new practice. We don't even have enough money
> to cover the children's college expenses now. I am deeply afraid
> that if he is accepted in the residency, I will be forced into the
> position of choosing between what is best for his mental
> happiness in his profession and what is best for our children's
> emotional and educational stability. Therefore, I have been
> forced to face the possibility of a separation. Needless to say, it
> isn't pleasant to face this situation. I don't think any choice I
> make in this situation will be a good one, because someone will
> be hurt no matter what action I choose to take.

These accounts convey a recurring theme in midlife, namely,
the need to make painful choices in which someone gets hurt no
matter what action is taken. As Rothstein (1980) pointed out, a
frequent midlife fantasy is starting over in one's personal life with
a new spouse and family, leaving the old problems behind. This
kind of thinking may lead to extramarital affairs and to divorce.
One physician's spouse said:

> In the last years of our relationship, I felt I was dying inside.
> What saved me was when I fell in love with a sort of flaky, wild,
> hippy, spiritual man. This relationship, while never sexually
> consummated, was the key to my realizing how incredibly alive I
> could feel in a relationship; and eventually it made me realize
> that I'd better get out of my marriage before I left with another
> man. My husband, whom I told, was furious, hurt, and never got
> over this. He definitely did not see this relationship as a sign that
> he and I should deepen our relationship as an antidote. He
> simply built his walls higher and stronger, and I think he never
> forgave me.

As this woman suggests, a new partner may seem to be the panacea for all midlife problems. Replacement is often much more attractive than mourning.

In other cases both partners are so fearful of having to live alone that they prefer to go on leading lives of quiet desperation. One physician described this feeling: "Living alone is a frightening alternative at my age; and, therefore, a loveless marriage but with mutual dependency and shared interest in children is to be borne. For brief periods it may even be mildly pleasant, and there are memories of happiness together."

Gillespie and Gillespie (1983) reported that in most physicians' marriages there is a strong tendency to deny dependency needs. Along with lack of intimacy and impaired communication, this may cause extraordinary difficulties at times of loss or grief. The death of a parent or the problems caused by a disappointing child often contribute to marital strife in midlife if the husband and wife do not know how to share the grief. Extramarital relationships are one way of trying to deny death and loss.

A certain type of hostile-dependent relationship is common. The traditional wife may insist that her husband is withholding nurturance and love, partly because she wants to avoid acknowledging that his emotional inarticulateness is the result of *incapacity*, not withholding. She thinks that intellectual prowess implies emotional competence, and sees silence as hostile and rejecting. Wives tend to label their experiences with such husbands "frustrating" rather than "disillusioning" or "disenchanting." The effort to maintain the illusion that the husbands will ultimately come forth with needed expressions of love reflects the psychology of postponement and confirms Robert May's (1980) observations on female fantasy. If postponement breaks down, the wife may face an agonizing choice. How much longer should she pursue a resistant, inexpressive, and affectively limited partner? At what point should she stop? Should she settle for less than she needs emotionally? It is far easier to avoid these painful questions and go on hoping against hope.

The Female Physician's Marriage

The female physician's midlife experience is different from the male's. In part this may be due to female psychology, but it is also partly because she has more options for creative solutions to midlife problems. She has probably not compartmentalized her life as much as the male physician. She is more likely to have been concerned with intimate relationships as well as work. As Gilligan (1982) pointed out, identity and intimacy are much more closely bound in women than in men. The female physician is therefore likely to enter midlife with a greater balance in her life than the male physician. This has a cost, however. Angell (1982) noted that in the female physician's mid-30s, the time of most rapid career advancement, she is also likely to be having and rearing children. Therefore she is not likely to achieve powerful positions in either organized or academic medicine.

Nontraditional women may have a fantasy script different from the traditional woman's. May (1980) reported one study (Saarni 1976) in which a group of "politically and organizationally active feminists" showed neither the female pattern of deprivation followed by enhancement, nor the male pattern of achievement followed by downfall. Instead, their scenarios represented pride and self-confidence without a disastrous ending. Certain competent professional women may be less prone to midlife decompensation because of a better synthesis of intimacy and identity throughout young adulthood.

Although the female physician is not likely to experience the same rude awakening as the male, the picture is not entirely rosy in midlife. Depression is common; more than half of female physicians may be diagnosable as having primary affective disorder (Welner et al. 1979). Even more alarming, the suicide rate of women physicians is three to four times that of women in the general population (Pitts et al. 1979). Often there is a crisis related to delayed childbearing and the biological clock. She must decide whether she wants a child or not. If she decides in favor, she must weigh the pros and cons of part-time work, full-time work, or staying at home with the infant. Any decision involves sacrifice, guilt, and anxiety. All female physicians are familiar with male colleagues who think they have cheated a man out of a slot in medical school when they take time off from work to have children.

Having a child is one way to deal with the midlife transition and even head off a major midlife crisis. However, the dual-career couple may now feel "out of synch." The husband despairs as he contemplates death and the limits of his youthful dreams; his wife is filled with joy and hope as she prepares for new life. Her husband needs more attention, but she is preoccupied with the baby.

Discussing the midlife transition in women would be incomplete without a word about menopause. Over the years menopause has been blamed for depression, hot flashes, night sweats, headaches, dizzy spells, palpitations, sleeplessness, weight increase, anxiety, and loss of sex drive. Studies do not support this; menopause is not a central event and not responsible for most symptoms (Notman 1979). Midlife stress in women results from various intrapsychic, interpersonal, biological, and vocational factors. Only night sweats and hot flashes are symptoms commonly linked with menopause. Depression results from loss of parents, friends, and children rather than from hormonal changes.

The woman in midlife must also accept the loss of her dream of being a perfect mother. She has not been able to fulfill the fantasy of correcting the mistakes she feels her mother made with her. The "empty nest syndrome" is often linked with midlife depression, but the "full nest syndrome" is also a source of stress. If the children will not leave home when they are expected to, the woman may have a sense of failure and feel guilty about setting limits on how long they can stay. In one variation of the full nest syndrome, parents and/or in-laws come to live with the chosen daughter, placing even more demands for nurturance on an already beleaguered middle-aged mother. Neugarten (1979) commented that caring for parents may create a more serious crisis in midlife than children leaving home or the loss of youth.

Positive Dimensions of Midlife Transition

While middle age may be a "dark night of the soul" for a great many physician couples, for others it is highly positive. Constructive mourning, reevaluation of goals, and consolidation of meaningful relationships occur. While licking the wounds to self-esteem inherent in realizing one's own mortality, the male partner can also benefit by reorienting his life away from career achievement and toward personal support and nurturance. One crucial shift is becoming a *mentor* (Levinson 1978) to children and younger colleagues; one can achieve a great deal of pleasure from seeing others respond to one's example. Serious reflection about existential issues such as the meaning and purpose of life also helps. As Nietzsche wrote, "He who has a *why* to live can bear most any *how*."

The marriage may reawaken in midlife. There is time to spend together alone without the children. Both husband and wife may feel free to come and go as they please without constantly placing the children's needs first. Many couples feel a stronger commitment, after going through difficult times with their children for many years. One physician's wife described such a transition:

> Our working through the problems that arose in the child-rearing years have created a commitment between us that, together with the support of family and friends, will see us through. Some of the areas of conflict would have been much higher when the children were at home. Since they are now away at school and doing a creditable job of managing their own lives, these sources of tension are no longer with us. We had considerable differences in child-rearing philosophy as related to discipline and methods. My husband was authoritarian with unrealistic expectations for performance, but with minimal actual involvement on a day-to-day basis. He had enormous professional demands and worked excessive hours. He believed all the hard work was for the benefit of his children, who weren't benefiting personally from his dedication. It has been a tough road at times and a slow evolution, but we've both learned a lot over the years. We've learned to observe and respect the generational dividing line. It may come through in other ways, but mostly we've learned to "keep our trap shut" and enjoy our children, their spouses, and their children for what they are. I worked for approximately 3 years full-time, and have satisfied my need for a career. I'm now quite content with my role as "just a housewife." Being married to a physician gives me the opportunity to pursue many outside interests. I consider myself very lucky.

The mourning process of midlife brings sadness, but also resignation and acceptance. Lowered expectations allow the spouses to enjoy each other for what they are. Many spouses no longer expect all their emotional and intellectual stimulation to come from the person they married. One middle-aged physician's wife described her situation in these terms:

> I think that basically we have a very solid relationship. Our backgrounds are very different; consequently, our insecurities are in different areas. Sometimes we struggle with communication; sometimes we're so close that there's no need for words; but in the long run, I think that's pretty human. I have structured my support system such that I can get what I need from several other people I am close to when I can't get it from my husband. So, though these periods are frustrating, they are not relationship threatening. We seem to be able to problem solve in most areas, which is something we have learned only in the last few years (and perhaps are still learning). We are deeply committed to one another and though periodically under great stress, I think we continue to grow.

The midlife crisis may well be a two-edged phenomenon, just as the Chinese figures for "danger" and "opportunity" combine to make the ideograph for "crisis." Even so, the midlife crisis is two-edged: a danger of serious depression, divorce, or catastrophic impulsive decisions, and an opportunity for rebirth and renewal.

In our survey (described in Chapter 2) we were quite impressed with the positive responses of middle-aged physicians. We divided the group into doctors and spouses younger than 43 and those who were older. There was no statistical difference in marriage gratification ratings, but there were signs that the older ones were more content. For example, older physicians talked to their spouses an average of 51.4 minutes a day as compared to an average of 32.8 minutes for the younger ones. Other statistically significant differences were as follows: (1) the younger physicians and spouses rated time away from home at work as a much higher source of tension in the marriage; (2) the younger physicians rated lack of shared responsibility for children and housework as a much higher source of tension; (3) the younger physicians more often complained that their spouses expected too much work around the house; (4) the younger physicians and spouses both rated lack of time for fun, family, and self as a greater problem; and (5) the younger spouses complained much more about their partners' lack of empathy.

This latter finding may reflect a greater empathy for others that often accompanies the aging process. When physicians acknowledge that they may never be chairperson of the department, editor of the specialty journal, president of the medical society, or the next Albert Schweitzer, they may then have more time and energy to devote to their families and social circles. The physician may share the experience of the spouse for the first time. We noted that men and women converge psychologically at midlife. This may cause a temporary asynchrony, but if both partners can adjust to a realignment of their relationship, there may be a more harmonious closeness.

Marital Therapy of Physician Couples

Stephen A. Jones, M.S.W.
Glen O. Gabbard, M.D.

Nearly half of the couples in the Chapter 2 survey sought marital therapy at some point, but most medical couples delay requests for help until the problems have become severe and entrenched (Krell and Miles 1976). Help may have been so long delayed that the marriage is unsalvageable, or can be saved only by intensive efforts over a long period of time. A decision to seek treatment may occur only when a crisis forces action. This crisis may take a variety of forms (or combinations of them): (*1*) a symptomatic husband or wife, (*2*) a symptomatic child, or (*3*) a problem involving both members of the couple.

In the traditional marriage, the problem often appears in the form of a "sick" wife. She may have mysterious physical symptoms, a major depression, a problem with drugs or alcohol, or a sexual symptom, such as inhibited sexual desire or anorgasmia. In a survey of hospitalized physicians' wives, Miles et al. (1975) found a high incidence of marital conflict. A physician suffering from depression, substance abuse, or (for males) impotence may be the first indication of a troubled marriage. Overwork to the point of exhaustion may reflect marital conflict. Sometimes physical illness brings latent marital conflicts to the surface. Because of physicians' tendency to rigidity and intellectualization, some authors suggest that the marital dyad is more likely than the individual physician to be amenable to therapeutic intervention (Glick and Borus 1984; Goldberg 1975; Krell and Miles 1976). Response to psychotherapy is variable; some physicians gain considerable relief from compulsive symptoms through psychoanalysis or individual psychotherapy. But individual approaches may not address the interpersonal issues of misperceptions and mutual disappointments that afflict a marital relationship. In fact, before the physician is able to change compulsive habits, the marital partners may first need to clarify and renegotiate their mutual expectations.

A marital problem may first appear in the form of an unmanageable teenager who manifests such symptoms as running away, drug and alcohol abuse, promiscuity, suicidal behavior, depression, poor school performance, or truancy of such severity that hospitalization is required. The general physician trained to diagnose individuals may see this problem as an example of individual psychopathology rather than recognizing such behavior as a symptom of an underlying family problem.

Infidelity is often the precipitating crisis. When one partner has been unfaithful, the other may see himself or herself as the innocent victim, and thus feel able to demand that both seek help. It may take a good deal of therapeutic work to help both partners understand that the affair is not simply an asymmetrical angry or impulsive act by one party, but the result of covert preexisting marital conflict. Departure of the children from home may move the couple to seek treatment by unsettling a tenuous balance in the marital relationship, or make evident a despairing emptiness in the relationship.

The Marriage Contract

The first step in marital therapy is a careful diagnosis of the difficulty. Sager's (1981) notion of the "marriage contract" is useful here. While contemporary couples occasionally write out formal contracts that they have carefully negotiated, Sager used the term to refer to a concept, rather than to an actual written document:

> Each partner in a marriage brings to it an individual, unwritten "contract," a set of expectations and promises, conscious and unconscious. These individual contracts may be modified during the marriage but will remain separate unless the two partners are fortunate enough to arrive at a single joint contract that is "felt" and agreed to at all levels of awareness, or unless they work toward a single contract with professional help. (p. 86)

Three elements of the psychological contract may be identified. The first deals with the *verbalized* aspects of the contract: issues and expectations that are openly discussed between the spouses, although what is spoken is not always heard and remembered. Secondly, there are *conscious but not verbalized* terms of the contract: feelings, expectations, and wishes not verbalized because of concern about the spouse's anger or disapproval. Thirdly, there are parts of the contract *beyond awareness or unconscious*, experienced as a passing sense of concern or a warning signal triggered in one's mind. A tendency to repeat entrenched patterns of relating to one another may also be part of the unconscious terms.

Verbalized Aspects

The verbalized terms are often explicit early in the engagement. For example, the male partner may make it clear that he expects to be the boss and that his wife will submit to his control. Many doctor–nurse marriages follow this model, in which the doctor's authority in the hospital extends to the home. A more extreme but still common variant is the doctor–patient paradigm of marriage.

> Fred and Ellen were one such couple. They were married just after Fred completed his residency in internal medicine. At the time of the wedding, Ellen had a serious alcohol problem. They explicitly agreed that he would always take care of her and treat her. He was careful not to take her to parties where alcohol was present, and he kept no alcohol in the home. He also prescribed Antabuse. When a major depression complicated her alcoholism, Fred prescribed antidepressants in addition. After almost 20 years of this less-than-successful treatment, Ellen finally decided that she wanted to enter psychotherapy to understand the underlying causes of her depression. Fred did not actively interfere, but he felt slighted by Ellen's suggestion that she needed treatment from someone else. They came to marital therapy when it became clear that the marriage might break up if Ellen changed as a result of treatment.

This example illustrates that the verbalized contract may fulfill an important homeostatic function although it may not meet all the unspoken expectations; attempting to alter it later may then disrupt the delicate balance of the marriage.

Conscious But Not Verbalized Aspects

The conscious but not verbalized terms of the contract may be the source of great resentment because each spouse often assumes that his or her partner should know these terms without being told. Each feels hurt and resentful when the partner does not live up to these unspoken expectations. Although this expectation that one's spouse should be a mind reader is patently absurd, it is a universal feature of troubled marriages.

As noted in Chapter 4, a physician husband very often feels that his wife should know exactly what his needs are after a heavy day of difficult practice, and how to gratify them without his ever having to make those needs explicit. He may come to feel more and more resentful if the needs go unmet, yet refuse to voice his expectations, partly because he stubbornly insists that his care, like care for a child, is her responsibility, and partly because having to ask for what he wants makes it seem less worth having or because asking exposes his unacceptable dependent wishes. Similarly, the wife may expect her husband to treat her in a particular but unstated way when they make love, and then resent his unresponsiveness to her unspoken needs.

> The case of Sam and Doris illustrates how the conscious but not verbalized terms of the marriage contract are often open secrets that both partners, by tacit agreement, never discuss. Sam, a radiologist, and Doris, a homemaker, came to marital therapy when one of their four children began rebelling at home and at school. The child was clearly Hispanic in appearance, although both parents were Caucasian. After several months, it emerged that many years ago Doris had had an affair with a Hispanic man, which she had never revealed to her husband. Obviously the child was not his, and though he had long suspected it, reference to the topic was taboo in the family.

Beyond Awareness or Unconscious Aspects

The aspects of the marriage contract that are beyond awareness or unconscious frequently involve expectations deriving from experiences in our families of origin. In choosing a wife or husband we are guided by earlier unconscious models of how parents and children behave toward each other or how our parents or siblings treated us, and we tend to seek out spouses who offer some possibility of fulfilling these unconscious expectations. A wife, for example, may implicitly expect that her husband will treat her very much like her father treated her mother. She may then unconsciously behave in a way that elicits this behavior. If, for example, her father repeatedly nagged her mother about failing to do housework, she may stop doing housework with the unconscious motive of provoking her husband to nag her about it. Sometimes the expectation is that one's spouse will behave in a diametrically *opposite* manner to one's parent. The husband, for example, may unconsciously expect his wife to behave in a manner that is in no way like his mother, with whom he did not get along. The wife may come to feel, without being able to say why, that in his eyes she never does anything right.

Marital Patterns

The marital therapist may observe significant behavioral patterns in the marital relationship. These patterns are distinctive "dances," characteristic styles of relating to one another that have become so habitual as to be almost automatic. Physician couples often fall into one of the five common patterns described by Murray Bowen (Kerr 1981): (*1*) conflict, (*2*) emotional distance, (*3*) triangulation, (*4*) overfunctioning–underfunctioning, and (*5*) pursuing and distancing.

Conflict

The partners overtly disagree, openly express disappointment with one another, often argue bitterly, and at times even fight physically. They may argue about everything: child rearing, sex, finances, in-laws, religion, power (i.e., who is dominant in the household), and responsibility for household work, as well as other seemingly trivial matters. But at least they are *engaged* with each other; they care about (or need) each other enough to put up a fight. If they give up fighting after years of stalemate, they may shift to the second pattern of emotional distance.

In dual-career couples much of the conflict centers on which spouse's profession comes first (Glick and Borus 1984) as well as the more familiar battles over responsibility for child care, housework, yard work, etc. As Berman et al. (1975) noted, despite lip service to the ideal of equality, there is often an underlying traditional stance of strong male–helpless female.

Emotional Distance

There is no overt conflict, but also no warmth, passion, love or verbal communication, and often no sex. Each partner suppresses difference or conflict, using the wish not to "upset" the other as a rationalization. This pattern can develop early in the marriage, but it usually evolves slowly over many years. The couple may finally come to marital therapy after having had virtually no communication or intimacy for 25 years. The marital therapist is confronted with the monumental task of reviving a dead marriage.

At this point in the marriage, some couples illustrate the mid-life crossover pattern (see Chapters 5 and 10). This crossover may accentuate a preexisting distance in the marriage. As they continue to lead separate lives, one or both may finally begin to look for other individuals or activities to meet their needs.

Many of these couples are not happy together, but remain married because they cannot imagine any alternative, and fear the loss of physical comfort and predictability. Sometimes they hope that the marital therapist can magically reignite the spark between them. This hope is usually unrealistic, so the therapist must help them choose between divorce or continuing deadness in the relationship.

Triangulation

In this pattern, the partners try to manage marital conflict by involving a third party. When a wife feels that her husband does not listen to her, she may use one of her children as a confidant instead. One chronically lonely surgeon's wife, who never complained to her husband, stated poignantly to her therapist that she had had a baby so she would have someone to love her. Triangulation of this kind can put a tremendous burden on a child. It is even worse when anger at a spouse is displaced onto a child.

A parent or parent-in-law may be triangulated into a marital conflict when intimacy is hard to achieve. Sometimes one partner does not separate from his or her family of origin. Later in the marriage, a live-in parent may serve as a buffer between the couple just as a child does.

Extramarital affairs are another form of triangulation. This attempted solution to the problem of an unhappy relationship may itself become a problem that requires another and more drastic solution.

Triangulation does not even require a third person. The practice of medicine itself has often been compared to a jealous mistress or, in Leichtman's words, a domineering in-law (see Chapter

9). Through overwork and prolonged absence, the physician may avoid an unhappy or threatening relationship at home.

Alcohol or drugs may also be involved in triangulation. One young resident who was addicted to meperidine (Demerol) went to elaborate lengths to hide this "affair" from his wife, also a physician. When he left the house to take the drug, it was like a secret meeting with a mistress. Because he knew that if he took a vacation with his wife, she would discover his addiction, for 3 years the couple never went out of town together. After extended treatment, he came to realize that he feared being alone with his wife and had used meperidine as a barrier to intimacy.

Overfunctioning–Underfunctioning

In this pattern, one spouse is dominant and the other submissive. The doctor–patient or doctor–nurse marriage often falls into this category. One spouse may also *overdo* to compensate for the other's lack of efficiency. One physician's wife reported that she went to bed every evening when her husband arrived home, explaining that she was exhausted from taking care of the children all day. Her husband would then make dinner for the children and help them with their homework to compensate for his wife's underfunctioning. On the other hand, a wife with an alcoholic husband may have to do twice as much work to cover up for her husband's drinking as well as to make up for what he is unable to do while he is intoxicated.

Pursuing and Distancing

This is a pattern in which one partner frantically tries to persuade the other to share more and spend more time together, while the pursued spouse works equally frantically to maintain the distance. This pattern is common in physician couples with traditional marriages, in which the traditional wife is a pursuer and the physician a distancer (Chapter 2).

> Fran, an obstetrician's wife, grew increasingly annoyed at her husband Jeff for leaving home without saying where he was going. Her husband sometimes even left town unexpectedly, calling her from another city to explain that he was consulting, teaching, or attending a conference. He wanted to be a "free man," he said. Resenting her insistence that he inform her of his whereabouts, he gave her less and less information. When he

discovered that she drove by the hospital to check on him, he parked his car two blocks away. One evening, tired of waiting at the supper table alone, she drove to his office, walked in, and discovered him partially undressed with his female bookkeeper on an examining table. That incident brought them into marital therapy.

Educational Interventions

It is often useful for the marital therapist to share his diagnostic understanding of the marital contract and patterns with the couple through educational interventions. The therapist may explain the concept of contracts and demonstrate how they operate in their marriage. Another useful intervention is to link the current marital pattern with larger patterns apparent in their families of origin (Kerr 1981). The therapist may help the partners see how they are unwittingly perpetuating styles of relating that span several generations. This helps them to feel less guilty about their own behavior and less accusatory of their partners. The marital stalemate can then be seen as a clash between two family systems, each trying to make the other conform to its own style. For example, triangulating third parties may be a well-established norm among parents and grandparents of one spouse, but wholly alien to the other. Family loyalties, rules, and expectations can be identified by means of these educational interventions, and a beginning sense of mastery on the part of each spouse may accompany this understanding.

Another type of education occurs when the therapist provides tools for better communication. The therapist may advise them that they will make their points better if they do not shout. They can also be advised to talk from the "I" position: Each partner is to speak only from his or her own feelings and thoughts and is precluded from blaming or accusing the other. The therapist may also give the couple home exercises to practice expressing their needs. This is the first step in teaching them to do *explicit contracting* instead of unrealistically relying on mind reading. The therapist may also urge the couple to learn to deal with disputes when they come up rather than store them away to be brought out all at once with a vengeance (in a tactic that some refer to as "gunnysacking"). Some couples find it helpful to have individual and marital developmental stages explained to them. This leads them to recognize the need to renegotiate their contract at each stage.

These educational interventions do not produce profound therapeutic change, but they serve an important function early in therapy. The physician couple usually comes to therapy at a moment of crisis, with emotions and accusations at a fever pitch. Teaching and explaining may diffuse the intense emotion by encouraging intellectual understanding and by allowing the couple to take a step back and contemplate the origins of their conflict in previous generations.

But more is needed to change entrenched patterns. The partners have reached their current state because it serves some important purpose for each of them. As a result, they are not likely to escape the impasse without a major struggle. Thus begins the next stage of marital therapy.

Resistances

Although both spouses proclaim their despair, the therapist quickly learns that neither is enthusiastic about change. Like superpowers in nuclear arms negotiations, the spouses feel that nothing important is negotiable and nothing negotiable is important. The enormously varied resistances to change are the focus of most of the therapeutic work.

Several authors (Glick and Borus 1984; Goldberg 1975; Krell and Miles 1976) have commented on one form of resistance: the physician's tendency to "play doctor" in marital therapy. For example, the physician may treat the therapist as an ally or colleague working as a cotherapist for the "sick" spouse. The physician may also compete with the therapist to make the most brilliant interpretations or the most ingenious therapeutic interventions, constantly arguing about theory and technique. The aphorism that good doctors make bad patients is highly relevant to marital therapy.

This behavior fits the classic definition of resistance: the emergence of a patient's characteristic defense mechanisms in the therapeutic situation. Physicians have spent their lives denying their own needs while catering to the needs of others. Doctors deny patienthood by taking care of others defined as patients (see Chapter 3). That is their defensive style at work and in the marriage, and the pattern continues in marital therapy.

George and Alice illustrate this situation. George was a psychiatrist and Alice a schoolteacher. They had been married 3 years and were emotionally committed to one another and to marriage as an institution. However, they had major sexual difficulties, which George viewed as Alice's problem. She had never experienced an orgasm with him or with her first husband. George tried to perform sex therapy with Alice as the patient. He was able to induce some sexual excitement through manual stimulation, but still failed to bring his wife to orgasm. He then prescribed a vibrator, which helped her to reach orgasm—but not when the couple made love. George approached the marital therapist as a colleague who would help him figure out a strategy for treating "Alice's problem." By this time Alice found the vibrator so much more stimulating than lovemaking that George felt quite threatened. The therapist pointed out that in most situations Alice felt that she was under George's control. Masturbating with the vibrator, *she* was in control. The therapist helped them redefine "Alice's problem" as a problem in the relationship. As George began to give up his need for control, Alice attained some control over her own orgasm, and was thus able to participate more actively in lovemaking.

Resistance to change may also reflect a hidden and largely unconscious agenda of thwarting the therapist's efforts. Each spouse may be secretly convinced that the other is at fault, and may feel disappointed when the therapist does not share that view. One or both spouses may resent the implication that they are partially responsible for their difficulties. They then undermine the therapist by refusing to follow suggestions.

The physician and spouse may also resist change because of a conviction that they do not deserve to be happy. One cannot underestimate the power of the physician's need for self-denial, self-sacrifice, and self-abnegation (see Chapter 3). Many physicians find their only source of satisfaction in hard work, long suffering, and masochistic self-neglect. When physicians get together, their faces light up as they trade "war stories" about their long hours, few vacations, and nights spent awake all night on call. The threat of improvement is that it might remove these comforting pillars of pain.

The person who marries a physician is also commonly a world-class sufferer. The physician's spouse knows what life will be like with a workaholic partner. Some traditional wives even glory in the bittersweet role of neglected, unappreciated martyr. At an unconscious level, they may enjoy making their husbands suffer by inducing guilt about their neglect. They also may have a strong investment in certain illusions or myths. An example is given in

Chapter 10: the wife who clings to the myth that her physician husband is withholding love, rather than his being unable to give it. Marital therapy may threaten to expose this myth by making it obvious that the husband has almost no capacity to express such feelings.

Change may simply be feared in and of itself: "Better the devil you know than the devil you don't." In physician couples this old saying may be particularly applicable to the fear of moving toward greater intimacy and commitment. For some there is comfort in distance. The prospect of an emotionally charged, frank discussion may represent an overwhelming threat. A case example nicely illustrates this dilemma.

Gilbert and Susan had been married 8 years when they came to marital therapy. Susan was somewhat depressed and had no interest in sex. The couple had not had sexual contact for the past 2 years. Susan wondered whether she had lost all trace of normal enjoyment in physical intimacy. They had enjoyed sex while courting, but sexual activity rapidly declined after marriage. As the treatment progressed, the therapist learned that through most of the courtship, Gilbert had been married to his first wife and carrying on a clandestine affair with Susan. Susan found the affair exciting and was impressed that Gilbert would take such trouble to be with her. Once Gilbert divorced his wife, much of the electricity went out of the relationship. The therapist pointed out to them that their original contract was based on a three-party arrangement designed to help Gilbert leave his marriage. When the task had been accomplished, the excitement was gone.

The therapist helped Susan to voice objections to Gilbert's treatment of her. She felt that he was emotionally unavailable, insensitive to her needs, distant with the children, and unwilling to help around the house. As Susan identified these issues and defined what she needed, she gradually became more sexually responsive. After 14 months of therapy, the couple had begun to resolve some of their differences. Susan became interested in affection and sexual contact again. But just when Gilbert and Susan had begun to enjoy lovemaking again, Gilbert had an affair with another woman while out of town at a convention and contracted genital herpes. He unwittingly infected Susan, and she reacted with rage and profound mistrust. All the painstakingly gained improvement was destroyed by this crisis. It took another year of treatment to restore enjoyable sexual and emotional intimacy.

When the intimacy of his first marriage disturbed Gilbert, he triangulated Susan as a possible solution. After their marriage they rapidly fell into a distancing pattern because the three-party arrangement was no longer applicable. When marital therapy seemed about to bring the couple into greater intimacy, Gilbert again felt threatened and again triangulated a third party.

The physician's resistance to intimacy can be formidable. Some physician couples drop out of treatment with a variety of excuses once the direction of the therapy toward greater intimacy becomes clear. With many couples, the marital therapist must be realistic about their limited capacity to change. It is necessary to be satisfied with some movement toward a more comfortable relationship, even though the intimacy achieved is far from ideal.

Gladys and Steve, both physicians, had been married 24 years. Gladys was most vocal about the couple's problems. She was angry and bitter about Steve's preoccupation with work and his insensitivity to her needs. She resented being entirely responsible for the household and child care even though she also worked full time. They had become quite distant when they finally came for help. In marital therapy, Steve acknowledged his failure to share responsibilities at home and slowly became more attentive to the children as well as to Gladys.

After a year of therapy, Gladys had become less bitter as she saw the changes in Steve. However, they continued to sleep in separate rooms, and Gladys continued to refuse sexual contact. She traced this sexual difficulty to an incident before their marriage in which Steve had casually walked by and dropped some contraceptives into her purse without discussion with her. She felt he expected her to sleep with him without his asking her if she was ready to make an emotional commitment to him. Gladys said she was uncertain about ever having sexual relations with her husband again. The therapy continued to focus on what Steve might do to help her feel more trusting and responsive. One day she came to the therapy session in a somewhat brighter mood than usual. She said that she had been troubled by some gynecologic symptoms the previous evening. Steve offered to give her a pelvic examination. She agreed, and afterward felt that Steve had passed the test by being gentle and caring. It was her way of allowing more closeness and trust in the relationship. Although their relationship improved emotionally, Gladys and Steve did not continue to work on their sexual problems. They ended therapy feeling that their lives were much better, but they also made clear the limits of change by deciding to cease all sexual contact and to sleep in separate bedrooms.

The therapist's neutrality is very important. Therapists must not be driven by a need to change the couple in any particular direction, nor even a need to change them at all. The therapist's role is to help them define for themselves whether and in what direction they want to change. Often the more one spouse pushes for change, the more the other spouse refuses it. The same principle applies to the therapist. If the therapist pushes hard for change, the couple will "circle the wagons" against an external threat, and their resistance will be heightened. Couples will assault the therapist's neutrality from all angles. Many will beg to be told what to do and then refuse to follow the suggestions. To maintain a neutral stance, the therapist must often simply present a variety of options; it is the couple's responsibility to choose one. Divorce is sometimes an acceptable outcome, and many therapists state this explicitly at the start so that it will not be seen as a therapeutic failure.

Change in Marriage

Change is primarily the responsibility of the couple, not the therapist. This may be a shock to physician couples who believe they have fully discharged their responsibility simply by coming for help. Each partner resists any effort to address his or her part of the problem. Each partner feels wronged; each expects substantial restitution. This self-righteousness often leads to a stalemate in which each expects magical change, chiefly in the form of a total transformation of the other. In the most favorable circumstance, the couple learns that the stalemate can be broken only through a painful process of concession, compromise, and recontracting in which each partner both gives and takes.

The therapist can encourage behaviors and attitudes that are conducive to change. Listening in an open-minded way without prejudgment is important. Understanding that one's spouse carries complex messages from a multigenerational family system may help a spouse to be forgiving and accepting. The spouses must be willing to reduce their investment in their own versions of "the truth." Flexibility and openness to new behaviors in one's spouse are also important. Each spouse can make a conscientious effort to recognize that there are several valid points of view on any particular issue.

Tom, a general surgeon, and Linda, a homemaker, had begun their marriage with an extensive verbalized contract. After marrying at the end of Tom's residency, they had agreed to live in the Midwest for 3 years and then move to the West Coast to be closer to Linda's family. In the Midwest Tom became increasingly involved in his practice; Linda became immersed raising three children and managing a household. When the 3 years were up, they continued to live in the Midwest, although they had had no new negotiations. Linda became angry and insisted they enter marital therapy, where she said she felt betrayed because Tom had not upheld his end of the bargain. She said he "beat around the bush" when she brought up the issue. After several sessions, Tom acknowledged that he remembered the agreement but said he was enjoying his job and did not want to leave. He had secretly hoped that Linda would forget his promise. With the help of the therapist, Tom and Linda started a renegotiation that led them to reconfirm the original contract. Tom found a job on the West Coast, and they moved within 6 months. Renegotiation brought them much closer together; in reaffirming their decision, they also reaffirmed the importance of their relationship.

Dan and Nancy were another couple who made good use of marital therapy. Dan, a chemical engineer, and Nancy, an oncologist, had been married for 13 years. They came to marital therapy because their 13-year-old daughter was becoming somewhat rebellious, and they feared she would get out of control. All three of them came to the first two sessions as a family. The couple showed up without their daughter at the third session and said that she had run off. Actually she had gone to a friend's house to allow the couple to come alone. It became clear that they had originally married because of Nancy's pregnancy, and had always felt embarrassed about their "mistake." They had always viewed their daughter as "illegitimate," although they had never discussed the ambiguous circumstances of her conception. They mentioned in passing that neither they nor their parents had ever formally acknowledged or celebrated their wedding anniversary. The therapist raised the possibility of renegotiating that contract. They acknowledged their collusion in maintaining the secret and began to allow changes in the family myths and rituals. Marital therapy helped them to see that it was their marriage that was illegitimate, not their daughter. As they "legitimized" the marriage, the daughter became much less symptomatic, and their own relationship more satisfying.

It is difficult to generalize about the outcome of marital therapy with physician couples. Goldberg's (1975) impression is that physician couples have somewhat better outcomes than comparable nonphysician couples. In the small sample of 15 physician families that Glick and Borus (1984) treated in marital or family therapy, they claimed a 92 percent improvement rate. Krell and Miles (1976) were less optimistic. The outcome depends, among other things, on how long they postpone seeking help, whether one or the other is in love with a third person, the willingness and capacity of each to change, and the presence or absence of individual psychopathology.

Since the spouse is both the physician's main support system and the first casualty of the physician's defensive strategy of overwork, the marital relationship is often the best level at which to intervene therapeutically when one or both partners become symptomatic. For those couples in less serious need, the tools for communication provided by marital therapy can also help the couple prevent future turmoil.

Responsibility for Self and Others: Improving the Medical Marriage

Roy W. Menninger, M.D.
Glen O. Gabbard, M.D.

Love is what you've been through with somebody.
—James Thurber

When a physician couple comes into marital therapy, they are acknowledging that they have not been able to negotiate workable solutions to their problems. Marital therapy, however, is certainly not a necessity for busy medical couples. More than half of the couples in our Chapter 2 survey had not sought marital counseling. Many medical marriages are creative and satisfying. These couples have learned how to cope with busy lives while also attending to each other's needs. From these couples, we have come to understand that it is vitally important to be aware of what *truly* matters to each partner and to be willing (and able) to talk about these issues.

It is commonly said that marital couples in trouble suffer from "poor communication." But at least as often, partners do not understand the underlying emotional issues that fuel the communication difficulty; they do not appreciate their own or their partner's needs. Male physicians especially seem not to know what they feel or how they hurt, let alone what may be troubling their spouse. Communication about such matters is limited or absent, or left by default to the more emotionally expressive member of the couple, usually the woman. Conversation between them often avoids touchy and emotionally important matters altogether. When pressures build and a fight breaks out, it is commonly over the wrong issue, or it is undertaken to establish the innocence of one partner and to attach blame to the other.

Emotionally successful couples know more about each other's "inner life"—not because they are more intuitive or more intrusive, but because they have developed some understanding of their own and their partner's emotional needs, and have found ways to share their common concerns. This vital awareness of personal needs is not automatic, nor even easy to develop through concerted effort. Developing it is the personal responsibility of each individual, not something a parent can or should do for a child, or one spouse for the other.

> Leonard and Madge's marriage exemplifies these problems. Madge, the physician, was the subordinate member of a two-physician practice started by her older partner, a motherly but dominating woman who had treated Madge as a beloved niece during her parentless childhood and adolescence. Madge found herself immobilized by guilt, unable to protest her senior partner's increasingly unreasonable expectations. Leonard, an attorney, had no trouble outlining clearly just what Madge should do and how she should do it. He experienced mounting annoyance at Madge's refusal to deal aggressively and forthrightly with demands that seemed excessive to him. He was quite unable to understand her special concerns. Madge felt annoyed at her husband's failure to see why she felt so constrained by a long-standing sense of obligation. The combined pressure of a difficult working environment and a husband who seemed to ignore her definition of what she needed was moving their relationship toward a stalemate.
>
> Leonard had his own need: to change the woman he had married from a feeling, empathic, and caring person into someone more like himself—focused, logical, systematic, and able to ignore the emotional aspects of a situation. He could not accept her needs as she defined them, but only as he felt those needs should be. Instead of helping her deal with her needs, he wanted to force a change in the needs themselves. The result was a power struggle and an impasse of mutual stubborn refusal to make any change at all.
>
> Change became possible only when Leonard recognized that he must not insist on Madge's compliance with *his* plans, and instead must simply raise questions that Madge might consider. As his pressure diminished, she felt freer to consider alternatives,

including more assertiveness at work. The issue here was not simply poor communication, but *what* was communicated. When he shifted from making demands to asking questions, their communication improved and the relationship grew.

To minister successfully to the needs of others and develop an emotionally healthy marriage, physicians must recognize and deal maturely with their own needs. Continuing to deny them guarantees alienation, withdrawal, affective flattening, decreased interest in other people, and chronic depression. Identifying and addressing these emotional needs is a central part of caring for the self. Yet most physicians hardly attend to their physical needs even when ill.

Their tyrannical consciences drive them to give first, last, and only priority to their patients. They have a self-image of invulnerability, denying the needs they attempt to meet in others (particularly in patients). Moreover, as we pointed out in Chapter 3, attention to one's own needs might upset a delicate defense designed to deny longing for nurturance and approbation, as well as suppressed anger about never having felt a sufficiency of either in childhood.

For thinking about the legitimate emotional needs of the self, there is no model to copy, no set of instructions to follow. The available models are bad ones. The rise of cultural narcissism (Lasch 1979) and the unattractive prominence of the "Me Generation" have provoked a reaction of unwillingness to acknowledge one's own needs to avoid seeming unpleasantly egocentric. Traditional religious and ethical teachings reinforce this tendency to identify thoughts about the self with self-centeredness and infantile self-indulgence. Yet we pointed out in Chapter 3 that narcissism per se is neither healthy nor pathological; it is pathological only if it interferes with efforts to balance one's own needs and those of others.

The path of least resistance is to avoid acknowledging the availability of alternatives. Most of us refuse to admit that we are *choosing* to continue living the masochistic and compulsive lifestyle of the typical physician. Ask any physician why he or she works such long hours, and the likely reply is, "I have no choice." To be sure, the events flowing from the original choice to become a physician can easily rob one of any further sense of choosing. But to deny that many small choices are still possible is to abdicate *all* sense of personal control. At the same time, to acknowledge that one's life-style *is* a choice is to face a painful reality. Therefore it is understandable, if regrettable, that, short of a crisis, most physicians and their spouses never pause to look systematically at their lives.

A Personal Review

We use structured queries to focus attention on habitual but unexamined behavior and thought, thus enabling people to see themselves in a new light. This involves challenging and necessarily broad and open-ended questions that are difficult to answer quickly or easily. The questions apply to the spouse as well as the physician, and so should encourage discussion between them. The questions call attention to concerns they have in common but may never have shared, and emphasize the gap between professed beliefs and actual behavior.

Goals and Objectives

The first of these questions is: What are your personal goals and objectives? Do you have any at all? Few individuals have thought much about this. The corporate world sees planning as vital to survival, but individuals do not. "Setting goals and objectives is something business people do, not me." For many, the perennial excuse of being too busy simply postpones the moment when the lack of a clear sense of direction and the absence of specific goals becomes an appalling reality—usually in the trough of a midlife crisis (see Chapter 10).

Even those few who do set goals usually concentrate on narrow economic questions such as life insurance, investments, and retirement benefits. Important work, to be sure, but stopping there leaves a huge gap. Most of us are not very concerned about failure to plan beyond the dollar sign. Again, we say we are too busy, but the message of our behavior is that asking pointed questions about our purposes and directions is not important.

Such questions demand that we assess what we are doing *now* and ponder the future consequences—a difficult and sometimes unpleasant task. Looking beyond tomorrow morning raises uncertainties and may cast doubt on decisions already made. It is easier to believe that the "future will take care of itself." And of course it will, if not altogether to our liking.

In part this is true because the many demands that the environment makes on us will continue to extract from us all we can give and, in so doing, force us to make impulsive, costly, short-term choices that may not take us where we'd like to go. But we do this mindlessly: We are on automatic pilot.

When physicians cite estate planning as an example of setting objectives, they illustrate a certain way of thinking about goals and objectives. Such thinking reduces goals to numbers that are intended to define our aims, our accomplishments, our progress, and ultimately our value as individuals. As measures of worth, an increase in such numbers is good because that presumably means an increase in value. Bluntly put, more is better; bigger is better.

When confronted with such statements, we chuckle as if to dismiss these remarks as absurdly simplistic and usually false. Yet we grudgingly acknowledge that we often think that way. Measures of quantity often insidiously metamorphose into statements of quality. Eventually these distorted standards are offered, and taken, as legitimate measures of achievement and even as the essential worth of others as well as ourselves.

Several years ago a young woman in California wrote a brief but eloquent essay about the perversion of values that accompanies the substitution of quantity for quality (Herbert 1977). It is a powerful caricature of our national preoccupation with numbers as the ultimate measure of quality.

The Snake: A Parable

In the beginning God didn't just make one or two people, he made a bunch of us. Because he wanted us to have a lot of fun and he said you can't really have fun unless there's a whole gang of you. So he put us in this playground park place called Eden and told us to enjoy.

At first we did have fun just like he expected. We played all the time. We rolled down the hills, waded in the streams, climbed the trees, swung in the vines, ran in the meadows, frolicked in the woods, hid in the forest, and acted silly. We laughed a lot.

Then one day this snake told us we weren't having real fun because we weren't keeping score. Back then, we didn't know what score was. When he explained it, we still couldn't see the fun. But he said we should give an apple to the person who was best at playing and we'd never know who was best unless we kept score. We could all see the fun of that. We were all sure we were best.

It was different after that. We yelled a lot. We had to make up new scoring rules for most of the games we played. Other games, like frolicking, we stopped playing altogether because they were too hard to score. By the time God found out about our new fun, we were spending about forty-five minutes a day in actual playing and the rest of the time working out the score. God was wroth about that—very, very wroth. He said we couldn't use his garden anymore because we weren't having any fun. We said we were having lots of fun, and we were. He shouldn't have gotten upset just because it wasn't exactly the kind of fun he had in mind.

He wouldn't listen. He kicked us out and said we couldn't come back until we stopped keeping score. To rub it in (to get our attention, he said), he told us we were all going to die anyway and our scores wouldn't mean anything.

He was wrong. My *cumulative all-game score is now 16,548* and that means a lot to me. If I can raise it to 20,000 before I die, I'll know I've accomplished something. Even if I can't, my life has a great deal of *meaning* now because I've taught my children to score high and they'll all be able to reach 20,000 or even 30,000 I know.

Really, it was life in Eden that didn't mean anything. Fun is great in its place, but without scoring there's no reason for it. God has a very superficial view of life and I'm glad my children are being raised away from his influence. We were lucky to get out. We're all very grateful to the snake. (p. 51)

The tyranny of numbers reinforces the tendency to define goals as predicates of two action-verbs: *having* (or acquiring or owning) and *doing* (or achieving or accomplishing). Goals characterized by such verbs are highly visible to oneself and to others; they are undeniable evidence of "worth." This readily combines with that unspoken belief that worth is appropriately measured by numbers, that more *is* better. A medical colleague recently spoke of his plan to write seven papers next year. Asked why seven, he replied, "Because I wrote only six this year." For that academic physician, numbers, not quality, was the ultimate measure. He apparently did not know (or wish to acknowledge) that his colleagues thought that five of this year's six papers contained nothing new.

One seldom hears a comment about goals and objectives that uses the verb *to be*. A male preference for action verbs may make it unsettling for some men to use the passive voice. Men are driven to achieve, to possess, to own, to control—all action-based verbs. But it may be more relevant to ask, "What kind of person do I want to *be*?" "What kind of person am I trying to *become*?" Put more cogently, how do we want to be remembered by our children (or, if it's too late for that, our grandchildren)? For many of us, at this moment at least, the answer is quite different from the reality: We're much too busy to stop and talk with them, let alone read them stories or take them for walks. Martin Buxbaum (1979) expressed this thought in a bit of poetic doggerel worth sharing:

> You can use most any measure
>   when you're speaking of success.
>
> You can measure it in fancy home,
>   expensive car or dress.
>
> But the measure of your real success
>   is one you cannot spend.
>
> It's the way your son describes you
>   when he's talking to a friend. (p. 56)

Priorities of Time, Money, and Energy

Closely related to goals are questions about one's personal priorities: Do you have priorities? Are they consistent with your behavior? Priorities in this context refer to the basis on which each person chooses how to use three vital resources: time, money, and energy. Conventional wisdom urges us to "set" them, or "establish" them, in the way a legislature creates a law or a judge renders a decision. The process is assumed to be straightforward; there is even an implication that those who don't or won't establish priorities are simply burdened with weak characters—a remnant of the volitionally based theories of psychological difficulties that were so prominent in the early years of this century.

There are many reasons for failing to set priorities, some of them more accurately described as excuses. To begin with, it is a difficult and complex undertaking. There are so many important issues, demands, and pressures, and the consequences are unclear. Many choices involve painful trade-offs; doing what we wish may extract a high price: guilt of our own or the anger of others.

As with goals, allowing others—one's family, one's colleagues, and especially one's patients—to determine priorities is one less-than-ideal way of setting them. Each makes demands for time and attention. Conscientious physicians often defer to the needs of others again and again, at the cost of repeatedly experiencing a diminution of self.

Physicians need less to set priorities than to examine them. Although they express choices in their behavior, that behavior may be inconsistent with their statements about what is important. Yet they are just as resistant to examining those choices as they are reluctant to set them in the first place, and for the same reasons.

For many of us, our use of these vital resources does not truly reflect our beliefs about what is important. Despite public protestations about the importance of the family and community, most of us devote little time to these areas. Many of us, especially the males, are married to our jobs, not to our spouses; we are invested in our patients and our colleagues, not our children; we are committed to our practice, not our society. Since this inconsistency is hidden by a morally irreproachable commitment to the ill, physicians are protected from having to recognize just how far out of balance their priorities are.

How people use time (in contrast with how they speak about it) illustrates their real priorities. For example, executives with broad responsibilities are presumed to use their time for the "big" issues, since that is how they typically describe their work. In fact, a careful study of their schedules may demonstrate that they spend much of their time on routine matters that others could handle (Drucker 1967).

Similarly, physicians are assumed to spend their time addressing issues of life and death, while in fact spending much of their time on matters of lesser importance, such as paperwork. Yet both executive and physician cherish the fantasy that their time is well spent and that they have control of it, oblivious to the contradictory truth.

This rather universal tendency is easy to demonstrate for oneself with the following exercise:

> On a blank sheet of paper, list the ways you spend time, ranking them in an approximate order of importance. The list must be an honest one, not a reflection of what things "ought" to be important or what other people might think. Then, on a second sheet of paper, develop a list of activities from a look at last week's schedule book and attempt a rough estimate of time spent doing each. Rank-order this list from largest to smallest. Then compare the second sheet with the first.

For most people, it is highly probable that last week's inventory will include few or none of the items on the list of "Activities

Important to Me." One may have spent the week having done very little explicitly defined as important. That discovery should shake some assumptions about one's planning and priorities.

People often explain away such omissions with reference to a very busy schedule, pressing deadlines, and the like, adding that they certainly will get to those important things "next weekend," or "next month," or "next year." They should live so long! Postponing is a common form of self-deception. It assumes we will have more time and opportunity tomorrow. Even more unreasonably, it assumes that we will be ready to do tomorrow what we haven't had time for today. Unfortunately, that usually happens only after a personal crisis such as a heart attack has captured our attention and forced us to do some fresh thinking.

Many cannot take seriously their list of important activities because doing so would reveal a distressing gap between wishes and actions. Keeping an action list that we do not pursue is testimony to one's good intentions, but it may be an example of modern "white magic"; its existence expresses a fantasy that "tomorrow," the happy and fulfilling reward that the compulsive workaholic seeks, will come.

Relationship to the Self

As we have noted, the self is a nebulous concept surrounded by complicated and contradictory feelings. To suggest an examination of one's relationship with the self is akin to suggesting passage through the eye of a needle.

Yet the effort is worthwhile. It is also possible if we think of the self as "a good friend" or "that kindly person in the next block," an abstraction free of the loaded connotations of "selfishness" and "egocentricity" that commonly afflict efforts to look at the self.

The central question to ask is how good a "friend" is the self? And following from that, how self-tolerant? How able to accept praise and appreciation? How ready to receive signs of love and caring from others?

The quality of one's caring for the self is immediately evident in one's expectations for performance. It is useful to ask whether one is willing to set *reasonable* goals for achievement, willing to acknowledge inevitable limitations and accept failures without converting them into new opportunities for self-criticism and castigation.

For many hyperconscientious people, the self is anything but a friend. It may even have become a kind of enemy: a barrier between work done and work that should have been done. Harsh criticism is aimed at this self; nothing is ever good enough; nothing ever fully measures up. Many effective and competent people would share Pogo's observation, "We have met the enemy—and they is us."

Excessively high and even unattainable demands on the self may result in remarkable accomplishments, but at a high cost. Falling short is more usual, but repeated failure rarely leads to a reassessment and modification of standards. The endless spate of criticism devastates normal pride in personal accomplishment and leads to chronic discontent and corrosive feelings of inadequacy. Sufferers burdened by high standards often expect others to do as well, and may even blame others (such as their spouses) for their own sense of personal inadequacy. This displacement of neurotic expectations complicates the relationship with both self and other.

When one takes seriously the image of the self as a good friend, strategies for appropriate self-care become clear. Even as caring for good friends requires time and effort, so does caring for the self.

An opportunity for play, for relaxation, for fun is part of caring for the self. Permission to enjoy without guilt is a potential antidote to the demanding, hypercritical conscience. Unfortunately, many physicians take this observation as a prescription. They respond by conscientiously scheduling time for relaxation and pursuing it compulsively, without ever noting the contradiction.

Permission for pleasure can often be given to the self only after sacrifice, pain, or discomfort. Dr. X. talked about the steps he follows in preparing for his vacation:

> First I must get *all* my paperwork up to date, even though this means working five successive nights until 2 a.m.; then I must be sure all the loose notes and papers piled on my desk have been properly filed or disposed of, and that I've left directions to my office staff and referral memos to the colleagues who will be covering for me that will anticipate every possible contingency that might arise while I'm gone. Then I set aside the articles and books I *must* get read while I'm gone, to be sure that every moment of my vacation time is well and fully used.

This man hardly knows the meaning of the word *play*, and his attitude is not exceptional. Another physician commented that he can have fun only when he makes work of it; unfortunately, giving oneself permission to enjoy without guilt is seldom sufficient. It may require years of psychotherapy or psychoanalysis before needs for self-punishment are sufficiently tamed to allow pleasure without guilt. Nevertheless, recognizing the pattern is an important first step.

Time should be devoted to endeavors designed to enrich one's life and the diversity of one's experience, and to broaden one's awareness of the environment. Time spent this way, and in doing some of the valued activities listed in the priorities test, is an investment in caring for the self. Enrichment challenges the constrictions of interest often entailed by the practice of medicine. To be successful, these caring activities require a personal commitment to *continued* growth, whether in knowledge, in competence, in perspective, in skills, or in experience. Those who continue to learn continue to live; those who don't have settled for a living death.

Successful caring for the self helps to move individuals closer to an ideal of emotional maturity (Menninger 1958, 1962):

- Having the ability to deal constructively with reality.
- Having the capacity to adapt to change.
- Having a relative freedom from symptoms that are produced by tensions and anxieties.
- Having the capacity to find more satisfaction in giving than in receiving.
- Having the capacity to relate to other people in a consistent manner with mutual satisfaction and helpfulness.
- Having the capacity to sublimate, to direct one's instinctive hostile energy into creative and constructive outlets.
- Having the capacity to love.

Strengthening the Medical Marriage

Responsible behavior toward significant others is a consequence of responsible behavior toward oneself. Thus a consideration of one's own values and goals will lead to a consideration of one's closest relationships.

Many of us fail to perceive how often our relationships are superficial, meager, and unrewarding, without real depth of emotional investment. It is too easy to attribute this lack to pressures and demands in our lives, the superficial materialism of the age, and so forth, avoiding any personal responsibility for the impoverishment that pervades our relationships.

Although the demands of medicine contribute to this impoverishment, the physician's difficulties with intimacy play an even larger part, as suggested in Chapter 3. Nonetheless, many medical marriages are satisfying and meaningful.

In such mature relationships, we have observed four prominent characteristics. We remind the reader that all of them rarely occur in an ideal form in any one marriage. Rather, they constitute an ideal toward which couples might strive.

A Spirit of Companionship

Nietzsche is alleged to have said, "It is not lack of love but lack of friendship that makes unhappy marriages." Indeed, many couples flounder when they fail to make the transition from being lovers to being friends. There are no substitutes for a sense of mutual trust and a reciprocal feeling of valuing and being valued. In the absence of such trust and liking, emotional growth is not likely, and the relationship is no more than an "arrangement."

Falling in love may seem effortless, but developing a friendship is not. It requires work. Most of all it requires time spent together in mutually enjoyable activity. This is a regular feature of the successful medical marriages we have seen. Husband and wife need time together that is both regular and inviolable. If they do not already have common interests, they can use this time to develop them. One couple made it clear to their children that Saturday night was "mom and dad's night," and none of the children's concerns was allowed to encroach on their time together. Both enjoyed a trip to the movies every Saturday night and discussion of the film afterward over dinner. Another couple found that their children's extracurricular activities and homework left no time for themselves. With considerable ingenuity, they worked out a way to meet for lunch three times a week to discuss their common interest in investment strategies.

Patterns of Communication That Honestly Express Individual Feelings

Making messages explicit is a healthy alternative to mind reading and inappropriate reliance on the infantile assumption that the other should understand without being told. But altering timeworn patterns of communicating is often difficult without help from third parties.

In healthy, vigorous marriages, communication patterns have several obvious characteristics. "Air time" is shared, with each listening as well as talking. Blaming and accusatory challenges are infrequent. Much of the affective communication is expressed in "I" terms, designed to share inner feelings and thoughts with the other. As a consequence, the capacity of each to empathize with the other is enhanced and the relationship strengthened. Appropriate humor helps to lighten intense feelings and permits both to gain distance and perspective on painful issues.

Shared Giving and Receiving

In some relationships, sharing is limited to tangible gifts or money. Mature giving addresses the need for psychological giving and receiving as well, such as in the communication patterns just referred to.

Negotiation is central to shared giving and receiving. In a mature relationship, both partners know they cannot always have their own way. In the "creative compromise" described by Bev Menninger in Chapter 5, each partner goes through a give-and-take process of bargaining. This negotiation is both verbal and behavioral.

> Paul and Carol were a married couple in their 30s who were quite satisfied with each other, although they acknowledged differences in their interests. Paul was a thrill-seeker who enjoyed risk and excitement; Carol was a conservative, cautious person who preferred the safety of home. They made concessions to accommodate each other's needs. Carol agreed to go snorkeling with Paul, and Paul expressed his appreciation by making every effort to make their snorkeling experience enjoyable. To Carol's surprise, she enjoyed it and suggested they do it again. Her willingness to negotiate and to take a risk led to a breakthrough in their relationship.

Shared giving and receiving means lowering expectations. Many high achievers believe that it is possible to have everything—especially professional women urged by the popular media to "have it all." Lowering expectations may be viewed as an admission of failure and therefore resisted. While characterological perfectionism may be difficult to modify, each spouse can help by giving permission to the other to stop short of idealized and un-realistic goals.

Attitudes about conflict illustrate this process. Couples in the Estes Park workshop repeatedly said that the family dinner was marred by disputes about the children's eating habits and mis-behavior, the irregularity of the meal, and so forth. Many couples seemed to feel that family dinners are so important that they should be ideally free of all conflict. Recognizing that this expec-tation is unrealistic may actually help to make meals freer of conflict.

One less obvious form of giving is a willingness to tolerate differences. We have already referred to pressures to "do things *my* way," "behave in ways that don't distress *me*," "be obliging and compliant to *my* expectations"—expectations that reflect a need for control, especially control over anxiety. Capacity to tol-erate individual differences that evoke anxiety is a mark of emo-tional maturity and psychological health. Giving here means noncontingent love, love that is not dependent on compliant be-havior.

Giving also means providing "strokes" and positive appre-ciation for the efforts or the words or simply the existence of the other partner. Protesting the charge that he did not often give his wife positive strokes, one physician said, "Of course I praise her! I don't criticize her when she does something wrong!" An inter-esting but hardly uncommon way of giving compliments. It is remarkable how often members of medical couples in our work-shop cannot remember when they last said, or heard, "I love you." One wife poignantly but doubtfully remarked that she thought her physician husband loved her because he had bought her the largest house in town more than 25 years ago.

One physician reported a chronic pattern of returning nightly to the hospital after dinner. Although his reasons were legitimate, his manner of taking leave from his wife often implied that he preferred his work at the hospital to spending time with her. In a painful confrontation with him shortly before she committed suicide, she said that she could have tolerated his absences more easily if he had managed to offset the negative implication of his departure with a suggestion that he would have preferred staying home.

Giving time to the other and arranging time together is an especially good indication of the value of a relationship; "lack of time" is nominally the main source of stress in medical marriages.

Passion

Each member of the couple must have room to express feelings and thoughts that may engage the other in vigorous, sometimes emotional exchanges—as long as they are focused and issue-oriented and not excuses for dumping accumulated resentments or accusations designed to defeat or utterly destroy the other.

Making Choices

The heart of personal responsibility is recognizing that we must accept "ownership" of the choices we've made, and see that improvement can only come from changes *we* make in ourselves and our behavior, not in others and their behavior. What most of us need is the incentive and the courage to reassess our choices and their costs.

Some costs are inevitable; there is no free lunch. The payee differs—not all are paid by the physician, some are paid by the spouse and family. The due date differs—not all costs are paid when incurred, many are a surprise when they come due years later. Physicians and their spouses can reduce these long-term costs with a close look at the impact of these costs on the self, the marital pair, and the family before it is too late. Making choices and assessing their costs requires:

- an honest examination of the values and attitudes that shape the choices the physician makes;
- a willingness to talk to others, and especially one's spouse, about them; and
- a readiness to seek alternative choices through negotiation and compromise.

Even then, balancing the demands of medicine with personal needs is not easy. There is no neat, clean, or permanent answer. No solution can be more than a temporary readjustment of a shifting scene. The dream of the young doctor described in Chapter 1—a harmonious and conflict-free balance between the medical practice and family life, with no residue of disappointment or failure—is indeed impossible. Given the importance of challenge to the human psyche, it is probably not even desirable. Emotionally mature couples will mourn the loss of youthful dreams and work to accommodate the vicissitudes of real life. The mature physician couple must strive *together*, persistently and creatively, to meet their own and their children's needs even as they retain a clear-eyed view of the requirements of the medical practice. The result will be growth for all.

Some years ago, Reinhold Niebuhr (1952) offered an eloquent perspective that is relevant to this Sisyphean task of balancing so many important, compelling, and unavoidable demands:

Nothing that is worth doing can be achieved in our lifetime; therefore we must be saved by hope.

Nothing which is true or beautiful or good makes complete sense in any immediate context of history; therefore we must be saved by faith.

Nothing we do, however virtuous, can be accomplished alone; therefore are saved by love. (p. 63)

Bibliography

Adsett CA: Psychological health of medical students in relation to the medical education process. J Med Educ 43:728–734, 1968

Angell M: Juggling the personal and professional life. J Am Med Wom Assoc 37:64–68, 1982

Anonymous: Equal, not really. JAMA 254:953, 1985

Anwar RAH: A longitudinal study of residency-trained emergency physicians. Ann Emerg Med 12(1):20–24, 1983

Barrand J: Masochism, masturbation and matriarchy: the doctor's family. Aust Fam Physician 8:663–667, 1979

Baruch G, Barnett R, Rivers C: Lifeprints. New York, McGraw-Hill, 1983

Bates EM, Moore BN: Stress in hospital personnel. Med J Aust 2:765–777, 1975

Bergman AS: Marital stress and medical training: an experience with a support group for medical house staff wives. Pediatrics 65:944–947, 1980

Berman EM, Lief HI: Marital therapy from a psychiatric perspective: an overview. Am J Psychiatry 132:583–592, 1975

Berman EM, Sacks S, Lief H: The two-professional marriage: a new conflict syndrome. J Sex Marital Ther 1:242–253, 1975

Bernard J: The Future of Marriage. New York, Bantam Books, 1973

Bernstein D: Women, psychiatry and surgery. Psychiatric Annals 7:92–100, 1977

Bibring E: The mechanisms of depression, in Affective Disorders. Edited by Greenacre P. New York, International Universities Press, 1953, pp 13–48

Biller HB: Father absence, divorce, and personality development, in The Role of the Father in Child Development (2nd ed.) Edited by Lamb ME. New York, John Wiley & Sons, 1981a, pp 489–553

Biller HB: The father and sex role development, in The Role of the Father in Child Development (2nd ed.) Edited by Lamb ME. New York, John Wiley & Sons, 1981b, pp 319–358

Bittker TE: Reaching out to the depressed physician. JAMA 236:1713–1716, 1976

Bowlby J: Attachment. New York, Basic Books, 1969

Bowlby J: Separation: Anxiety and Anger. New York, Basic Books, 1973

Brazelton TB: Infants and Mothers. New York, Dell, 1969

Brazelton TB: Toddlers and Parents: A Declaration of Independence. New York, Delacorte Press, 1974

Brazelton TB, Als H: Four early stages in the development of mother-infant interaction. Psychoanal Study Child 34:349–370, 1979

Brim OG: Theories of the male mid-life crisis. Counseling Psychologist 6:2–9, 1976

Buxbaum M: Untitled. Reader's Digest, April 1979, p 56

Callan JP (ed): The Physician: A Professional Under Stress. Norwalk, Conn, Appleton-Century-Crofts, 1983

Cartwright LK: Conscious factors entering into decisions of women to study medicine. Journal of Social Issues 28:201–215, 1972a

Cartwright LK: Personality differences in male and female medical students. Psychiatry in Medicine 3:213–218, 1972b

Cartwright LK: Personality/family background, University of California female medical students. J Am Med Wom Assoc 27:5, 260, 1972c

Colarusso CA, Nemiroff RA: Some observations and hypotheses about the psychoanalytic theory of adult development. Int J Psychoanal 60:59–71, 1979

Coombs RH: The medical marriage, in Psychological Aspects of Medical Training. Edited by Coombs RH, Vincent CE. Springfield, Ill, Charles C Thomas, 1971

Crawford LE, Lorch BD: Physician's wives: an examination of their place in the stratification system. Social Science Journal 18:69–80, 1981

Derdeyn AP: The physician's work and marriage. Int J Psychiatry Med 9:297–306, 1978

Drucker P: The Effective Executive. New York, Harper & Row, 1967

Duki WG: Study of medical school students. J Med Educ 46:837–857, 1971

Eisenberg L: Distaff of Aesculapius—the married woman as physician. J Am Med Wom Assoc 36:84–88, 1981

Elliot FR: Professional and family conflicts in hospital medicine. Social Science and Medicine [A] 13:57–64, 1979

Emde RN: Toward a psychoanalytic theory of affect, II. emerging models of emotional development in infancy, in The Course of Life, Vol. 1. Edited by Greenspan SI, Pollock GH. Washington, Department of Health and Human Services, 1980

Emde RN, Robinson J: The first two months: recent research in developmental psychobiology and the changing view of the newborn, in Basic Handbook of Child Psychiatry, Vol. 1. Edited by Noshpitz JD. New York, Basic Books, 1979, pp 72–105

Epstein C: Encountering the male establishment: sex-status limits on women's careers in the professions. American Journal of Sociology 15:6–9, 1975

Erikson EH: Childhood and Society. New York, WW Norton, 1963

Erikson EH: Identity, Youth, and Crisis. New York, WW Norton & Co, 1968

Evans JL: Psychiatric illness in the physician's wife. Am J Psychiatry 122:159–163, 1965

Fine C: Married to Medicine: An Intimate Portrait of Doctors' Wives. New York, Atheneum, 1981

Frank E, Anderson C, Rubinstein D: Frequency of sexual dysfunction in "normal" couples. N Engl J Med 299:111–115, 1978

Freud S: The interpretation of dreams (1900), in Complete Psychological Works. Standard Edition, Vols. 4 & 5. Translated and edited by Strachey J. London, Hogarth Press, 1962

Fruen M, Rothman A, Steiner J: Comparison of characteristics of male and female medical school applicants. J Med Educ 49:137–145, 1974

Gabbard G: The role of compulsiveness in the normal physician. JAMA 254:2926–2929, 1985

Gaddy C, Glass C, Arnkoff D: Career involvement of women in dual-career families: the significance of sex role identity. Journal of Counseling Psychology 320:388–394, 1983

Garvey M, Tuason VB: Physician marriages. J Clin Psychiatry 40:129–131, 1979

Gerber LA: Married to Their Careers: Career and Family Dilemmas in Doctors' Lives. New York, Tavistock, 1983

Gillespie HG, Gillespie CL: The divorced physician: autopsy of a medical marriage, in The Physician: A Professional Under Stress. Edited by Callan JP. Norwalk, Conn, Appleton-Century-Crofts, 1983, pp 150–166

Gilligan C: In a Different Voice. Cambridge, Mass, Harvard University Press, 1982

Glick ID, Borus JF: Marital and family therapy for troubled physicians and their families: a bridge over troubled waters. JAMA 251:1855–1858, 1984

Goldberg, M: Conjoint therapy of male physicians and their wives. Psychiatric Opinion 12(4):19–23, 1975

Gove WR, Tudor JF: Adult sex roles and mental illness. American Journal of Sociology 78:812–835, 1973

Gutmann D: An exploration of ego configurations in middle and later life, in Personality in Middle and Late Life. Edited by Neugarten B. New York, Atherton Press, 1964, pp 114–148

Hall R, Sandler B: The classroom climate: a chilly one for women? (Project on the Status and Education of Women) Washington, DC, Association of American Colleges, 1982

Heinicke CM: Development from two and one-half to four years, in Basic Handbook of Child Psychiatry, Vol. 1. Edited by Noshpitz JD. New York, Basic Books, 1979, pp 167–178

Heins M, Smock S, Martindale L, et al.: Comparison of the productivity of women and male physicians. JAMA 237:2514–2517, 1977a

Heins M, Smock S, Martindale L, et al.: A profile of the woman physician. J Am Med Wom Assoc 32:421–427, 1977b

Herbert A: The snake: a parable. The CoEvolution Quarterly 13:51, March 27, 1977

Hiller DV, Philliber WW: Predicting marital and career success among dual-worker couples. Journal of Marriage and the Family 44:53–62, 1982

Horner M: Toward an understanding of achievement-related conflicts in women. Journal of Social Issues 28:157–175, 1972

Jacobson E: The Self and the Object World. New York, International Universities Press, 1964

Jaques E: Death and the mid-life crisis. Int J Psychoanal 46:502–514, 1965

Johnson SJ: Understanding dual-career couples. Cited by Parker M, Peltier S, Wolleat P. Personal Guidance Journal 60:14–18, 1981

Jones L: Why women execs stop before the top. Cited in Brophy B with Linnon N, U.S. News and World Report 10(26):72–73, December 29, 1986/January 5, 1987

Jussim J, Muller C: Medical education for women: how good an investment? J Med Educ 50:571–581, 1975

Kasper A: The doctor and death, in The Meaning of Death. Edited by Feifel H. New York, McGraw-Hill, 1959, pp 259–270

Kelner M, Rosenthal C: Postgraduate medical training, stress and marriage. Can J Psychiatry 31:22–24, 1986

Keniston K: The medical student. Yale J Biol Med 39:346–356, 1967

Kerr M: Family systems theory and therapy, in Handbook of Family Therapy. Edited by Gurman A, Kniskern D. New York, Brunner/Mazel, 1981, pp 226–264

Kilpatrick AC: Job change in dual-career families: danger or opportunity? Family Relations 31:363–368, 1982

Kimball C: Medical education as a humanizing process. J Med Educ 48:71–77, 1973

Kosa J, Coker RE Jr: The female physician in public health: conflict and reconciliation of the sex and professional roles. Sociology and Social Research 49:294–305, 1965

Krakowski AJ: Doctor-doctor relationship. Psychosomatics 12:11–15, 1971

Krakowski AJ: Stress and the practice of medicine: II. stressors, stresses, and strains. Psychother Psychosom 38:11–23, 1982

Krakowski AJ: Stress and the practice of medicine: III. physicians compared with lawyers. Psychother Psychosom 42:143–151, 1984

Krell R, Miles J: Marital therapy of couples in which the husband is a physician. Am J Psychother 30:267–275, 1976

Lamb ME (ed): The Role of the Father in Child Development. New York, John Wiley & Sons, 1976

Lamb ME (ed): The Role of the Father in Child Development (2nd ed.) New York, John Wiley & Sons, 1981

Lasch C: The Culture of Narcissism. New York, WW Norton & Co, 1979

Levinson D: The Seasons of a Man's Life. New York, Alfred A Knopf, 1978

Linn LS, Yager J, Cope D, et al.: Health status, job satisfaction, job stress, and life satisfaction among academic and clinical faculty. JAMA 254:2775–2782, 1985

Lopate C: Women in Medicine. Baltimore, Johns Hopkins University Press, 1968

Maccoby E, Jacklin C: The Psychology of Sex Differences. Stanford, Calif, Stanford University Press, 1974

Mahler MS, Pine F, Bergman A: The Psychological Birth of the Human Infant: Symbiosis and Individuation. New York, Basic Books, 1975

Malmquist CP: Development from thirteen to sixteen years, in Basic Handbook of Child Psychiatry, Vol. 1. Edited by Noshpitz JD. New York, Basic Books, 1979, pp 205–213

Masters W, Johnson V: Human Sexual Inadequacy. Boston, Little, Brown & Co, 1970

Mawardi BH: Satisfactions, dissatisfactions and causes of stress in medical practice. JAMA 241:1483–1486, 1979

May R: Sex and Fantasy: Patterns of Male and Female Development. New York, WW Norton & Co, 1980

McClinton JB: The doctor's own wife. Can Med Assoc J 47:472–476, 1942

McCranie EW, Hornsby JL, Calvert GC: Practice and career satisfaction among residency trained family physicians: a national survey. J Fam Pract 14:1107–1114, 1982

McCue JD: The effects of stress on physicians in their medical practice. N Engl J Med 306:458–463, 1982

McGrath E, Zimet C: Sex differences in specialty attitudes and personality among medical students, and their implications. Proceedings of Fifteenth Annual Conference of AAMC on Research in Medical Education, San Francisco, November 1976

Mechanic D: The organization of medical practice and practice orientations among physicians in prepaid and nonprepaid primary care settings. Med Care 13:189–204, 1975

Menninger KA: Psychological factors in the choice of medicine as a profession, part II. Bull Menninger Clin 21:99–106, 1957

Menninger WC: Growing up emotionally, in Blueprint for Teen-age Living. Edited by Menninger WC. New York, Sterling Publishing Co, 1958, pp 5–49

Menninger WC: Seven keys to a happy life. Address reprinted in Des Moines Sunday Register, 7 October 1962

Miles JE, Krell R, Lin T: The doctor's wife: mental illness and marital pattern. Int J Psychiatry Med 6:481–487, 1975

Money J, Ehrhardt A: Man and Woman: Boy and Girl. Baltimore, Johns Hopkins University Press, 1972

Moore K, Spain D, Bianchi S: Working wives and mothers. Marriage and Family Review 7:77–98, 1987

Nadelson C: The woman physician: past, present and future, in The Physician: A Professional Under Stress. Edited by Callan JP. Norwalk, Conn, Appleton-Century-Crofts, 1983, pp 261–276

Nadelson C, Nadelson T: The dual-career family, in Modern Perspectives in Psycho-Social Pathology. Edited by Howells J. New York, Brunner/Mazel, 1988

Nadelson C, Notman M: Adaptation to stress in physicians, in Becoming a Physician. Edited by Shapiro E, Lowenstein L. Cambridge, Mass, Ballinger, 1979

Nadelson C, Notman M, Lowenstein P: The practice patterns, life styles, and stresses of women and men entering medicine: a follow-up study of Harvard Medical School graduates from 1967 to 1977. J Am Med Wom Assoc 34:400–406, 1979

Nelson SB: Some dynamics of medical marriages. J R Coll Gen Prac 28:585–586, 1978

Neugarten BL: Toward a psychology of the life cycle, in Middle Age and Aging. Edited by Neugarten B. Chicago, University of Chicago Press, 1968, pp 137–147

Neugarten BL: Time, age, and the life cycle. Am J Psychiatry 136:887–894, 1979

Niebuhr R: The Irony of American History. New York, Charles Scribner's Sons, 1952

Notman M: Midlife concerns of women: implications of the menopause. Am J Psychiatry 136:1270–1274, 1979

Notman M, Nadelson C: Medicine: a career conflict for women. Am J Psychiatry 130:1123–1127, 1973

Notman M, Nadelson C, Bennett M: Achievement conflict in women: psychotherapeutic considerations. Psychother Psychsom 29:203–213, 1978

Notman M, Salt P, Nadelson C: Stress and adaptation in medical students: who is most vulnerable? Compr Psychiatry 25:355–366, 1984

Offer D, Offer JB: From Teenage to Young Manhood: A Psychological Study. New York, Basic Books, 1975

Osherson S, Dill D: Varying work and family choices: their impact on men's work satisfaction. Journal of Marriage and the Family 45:339–346, 1983

Ottenberg P: The "physician's disease": success and work addiction. Psychiatric Opinion 12(4):6–11, 1975

Owens A: Is medical practice a marriage breaker? Medical Economics 43:68–78, 1966

Perun PJ, Del Vento Bielby D: Towards a model of female occupational behavior: a human development approach. Psychology of Women Quarterly 6:234–252, 1981

Petersen AC, Offer D: Adolescent development: sixteen to nineteen years, in Basic Handbook of Child Psychiatry, Vol. 1. Edited by Noshpitz JD. New York, Basic Books, 1979, pp 213–233

Phelps CE: Women in American medicine. J Med Educ 43:916–924, 1968

Pitts FN Jr, Schuller AB, Rich CL, et al.: Suicide among US women physicians, 1967-1972. Am J Psychiatry 136:694–696, 1979

Pollak S, Gilligan C: Images of violence in Thematic Apperception Test stories. J Pers Soc Psychol 42:159–167, 1982

Powell GJ: Psychosocial development: eight to ten years, in Basic Handbook of Child Psychiatry, Vol. 1. Edited by Noshpitz JD. New York, Basic Books, 1979, pp 190–199

Powers L, Parmelle RD, Wiesenfelder H: Practice patterns of women and men physicians. J Med Educ 44:481–491, 1969

Rank O: Beyond Psychology (1941). New York, Dover Books, 1958

Renshaw DC: Recognition and treatment of sexual disorders. Penn Med, 86:1, 64–67, 1983

Rhoads J: Overwork. JAMA 237:2615–2618, 1977

Rose KD, Rosow I: Marital stability among physicians. California Medicine 16:95–99, 1972

Rothstein A: The Narcissistic Pursuit of Perfection. New York, International Universities Press, 1980

Saarni C: Social-cohort effect on three masculinity-femininity instruments and self-report. Psychol Reports 38:1111–1118, 1976

Sager CJ: Couples therapy and marriage contracts, in Handbook of Family Therapy. Edited by Gurman A, Kniskern D. New York, Brunner/Mazel, 1981, pp 85–130

Salsberger AB, Marder WD, Willke RJ: Practice characteristics of male and female physicians. Data Watch, Health Affairs 6:104–109, 1987

Sargent DA: Quoted in Major loss tied to eighty-five percent of MD suicides. Clinical Psychiatry News 13(7):3, 1985

Sargent DA: Quoted in Characteristics of physician at risk for suicide cited. Clinical Psychiatry News 14(4):20, 1986

Sayres M, Wyshak G, Denterlein G, et al.: Pregnancy during residency. N Engl J Med 314:418–423, 1986

Scarf M: Unfinished Business: Pressure Points in the Lives of Women. Garden City, NY, Doubleday & Co, 1980

Scarlett EP: Doctor out of Zebulun: the doctor's wife. Arch Intern Med 115:351–357, 1965

Schoicket S: The physician's marriage. J Med Soc NJ 75:149–152, 1978

Shaw J: The physician's marriage, II: the practice years. Facets 42:21–24, 1985

Shortt SED: Psychiatric illness in physicians. Can Med Assoc J 121:283–288, 1979

Silverman MA, Rees K, Neubauer PB: On a central psychic constellation. Psychoanal Study Child 30:127–157, 1975

Smith CS: Doctors' Wives: The Truth About Medical Marriages. New York, Seaview Books, 1980

Solnit AJ: Psychosexual development: three to five years, in Basic Handbook of Child Psychiatry Vol. 1. Edited by Noshpitz JD. New York, Basic Books, 1979, pp 178–184

Spitz RA: The First Year of Life: A Study of Normal and Deviant Development of Object Relations. New York, International Universities Press, 1965

Steppacher RC, Mausner JS: Suicide in male and female physicians. JAMA 228:323–328, 1974

Stern DN: The First Relationship: Infant and Mother. Cambridge, Mass, Harvard University Press, 1977

Stern DN: The Interpersonal World of the Infant. New York, Basic Books, 1985

Stoller RJ: Overview: the impact of new advances in sex research on psychoanalytic theory. Am J Psychiatry 130:241–251, 1975

Taubman RE: Medical marriages, in Marital and Sexual Counseling in Medical Practice. Edited by Abse DW, Nash EM, Louden LMR. Hagerstown, Md, Harper & Row, 1974

Taylor AD, Taylor RB, Taylor DM, et al.: Marriage, medicine, and the medical family, in The Physician: A Professional Under Stress. Edited by Callan JP. Norwalk, Conn, Appleton-Century-Crofts, 1983, pp 5–27

Terhune WB: The doctor's wife: "the acolyte of medicine." Conn State Med J 11:576–581, 1947

Terman LM: Scientists and non-scientists in a group of 800 gifted men. Psychological Monographs 68:1–44, 1954

Thomas CB: What becomes of medical students: the dark side. Johns Hopkins Medical Journal 138:185–195, 1976

Vaillant GE, Sobowale NC, McArthur C: Some psychological vulnerabilities of physicians. N Engl J Med 287:372–375, 1972

Vincent MO: Doctor and Mrs.—their mental health. Canadian Psychiatric Association Journal 14:509–15, 1969

Waring EM: Psychiatric illness in physicians: a review. Compr Psychiatry 15:519–530, 1974

Weinberg E, Rooney J: Performance of female medical students. J Med Educ 48:240, 1973

Weissman MM, Klerman GL: Sex differences and the epidemiology of depression. Arch Gen Psychiatry 34:98–111, 1977

Weitzman LJ: The Divorce Revolution, the Unexpected Social and Economic Consequences for Women and Children in America. Stanford, Calif, Stanford University Press, 1985

Welner A, Marten S, Wochnick E, et al.:Psychiatric disorders among professional women. Arch Gen Psychiatry 36:169–179, 1979

Wilson WP, Larson DB: The physician and spouse. NC Med J 42:106–109, 176–180, 274–277, 1981

Wolf MH: How to Be a Doctor's Wife Without Really Dying. Sarasota, NY, Booklore Publishers, 1978

Zabarenko RN, Zabarenko L, Pittenger RA: The psychodynamics of physicianhood. Psychiatry 33:102–118, 1970

Zemon-Gass G, Nichols, WC: "Take me along"—a marital syndrome. Journal of Marriage and Family Counseling 1:209–217, 1975

Index